BISPHOSPHONATES
IN BONE DISEASE

DEDICATION

To

My wife Maria Pia

My children Marie-Gabrielle, Isabelle Désirée and Marie-Laure

My father Alfred Fleisch who taught me scientific thinking and experimental rigor

William F. Neuman who introduced me to the bone

BISPHOSPHONATES
IN BONE DISEASE
From the laboratory to the patient

Second Edition

Herbert Fleisch MD

Professor and Head
Department of Pathophysiology
University of Berne
Berne, Switzerland

The Parthenon Publishing Group
International Publishers in Medicine, Science & Technology

NEW YORK   LONDON

Published in the UK by
The Parthenon Publishing Group Ltd.
Casterton Hall
Carnforth, Lancs LA6 2LA, England

Published in North America by
The Parthenon Publishing Group Inc.
One Blue Hill Plaza
New York 10965, USA

British Library Cataloguing in Publication Data

Fleisch, Herbert
  Bisphosphonates in Bone Disease: From the
  Laboratory to the Patient. – 2 Rev.ed
  I. Title
  616.71061

Library of Congress Cataloging-in-Publication Data

Fleisch, Herbert.
    Bisphosphonates in bone disease : from the laboratory to the patient / Herbert
  Fleisch.—2nd ed.
       p.   cm.
    Includes bibliographical references and index.
    ISBN 1-85070-705-7
      1. Diphosphonates—Therapeutic use.   2. Bones—Diseases—Chemotherapy.
  3. Calcium—Metabolism—Disorders—Chemotherapy.
  I. Title.
      [DNLM: 1. Bone Diseases—drug therapy.   2. Bone Diseases—metabolism.
  3. Diphosphonates—therapeutic use.   4. Diphosphonates—pharmacology.
  WE 225 F596b 1995]
  RC930.F54   1995
  616.7'1061—dc20
  DNLM/DLC
  for Library of Congress   95-37749
                                                                                  CIP

Hardback edition: ISBN 1-85070-705-7
Paperback edition: ISBN 1-85070-729-4

The cover illustrations were reproduced with the kind permission of Professor Boyde,
Department of Biology and Medicine, University College, London, UK

Typeset by AMA Graphics Ltd, Preston, Lancs
Printed and bound in Great Britain by Butler & Tanner Ltd., Frome and London

Contents

Note: The arrows which appear in the margins (➔) indicate the text to which the reader is referred by the captions, also in the margins.

Contents

Preface

The bisphosphonates are a new class of drug which have been developed in the past three decades for use in various diseases of bone and calcium metabolism. Five are commercially available today. Those available, as well as the indications for which they are registered, vary from country to country. A substantial number are under preclinical or clinical development, so that in the near future specialists and practitioners will have the opportunity to choose the most suitable drug and the best regimen to treat an individual patient.

Information for the doctor is available today in original articles, in a few reviews and in the documentation distributed by the companies selling the various compounds. No complete, easy to read publication in which the practicing doctor can quickly find the necessary information on all bisphosphonates has been available so far. This book has been written to cover this deficit.

It starts with a chapter giving a small *aperçu* of the physiology of bone. It then covers, in the preclinical part, the chemistry, mechanisms of action and animal toxicology of these compounds. In the clinical part, before addressing the use of the bisphosphonates, the diseases treated by these compounds are briefly discussed with respect to their pathophysiology, clinical picture and treatment with other drugs. After a chapter on adverse events, the book ends with a table containing the trade names of the commercially available bisphosphonates, the registered indications and the available forms for each country.

In order to keep this booklet concise, it was necessary to simplify many of the issues and therefore to make choices. It is hoped that the result nevertheless represents faithfully the state of the art. Literature had to be kept very restricted, the reader being referred when possible to reviews for further information.

I would like to express here my gratitude to Professor W.F. Neuman, Radiation Biology Department, Rochester NY, USA, where the seeds of this work were planted, to Professor A. Fleisch, Professor M. Allgöwer, Professor M.E. Müller and the Canton of Berne who gave me the possibility to pursue and develop this research in the Department of Physiology of the University of Lausanne, the Laboratory for Experimental Surgery, Davos, and the Department of Pathophysiology of the University of Berne.

I also thank Dr M.D. Francis with whose collaboration the bisphosphonates were born, my collaborators over these many years, who have allowed an idea to become reality, and my colleagues M. Cecchini, P.D. Delmas, J.A. Kanis, T.J. Martin, J.P.J. Meunier, S.E. Papapoulos, R. Rizzoli, G.A. Rodan, R.K. Schenk and D. Thiébaud, who have read and improved various parts of this work, and V. Antic for drawing some of the slides. Also, we are grateful to Dr Alan Boyde for providing the figures for the cover.

The first edition appeared in 1993. Since then an Italian version has published and a Japanese one is in print. In view of the rapid development in this field, it appeared adequate to prepare an updated second English edition. All chapters have been retained; some of them, such as those on Paget's disease and osteoporosis, extensively amended. While the first edition was exclusively distributed by pharmaceutical companies interested in the field, this one is also available in bookshops with the aim of making it available to a larger public worldwide.

September 1995   Herbert Fleisch

1. Bone and mineral metabolism

1.1. BONE PHYSIOLOGY

1.1.1. Morphology

Macroscopically, bone can be divided into an outer part called cortical or compact bone, which makes about 70% of the total skeleton, and an inner part named cancellous, trabecular, or spongy bone. This structure, an outer cortical sheath and an inner three-dimensional trabecular network, allows optimal mechanical function with minimal weight.

Biomechanical adaptation p. 26

> *Bone is a superb engineering construction with an outer compact sheath and an inner trabecular scaffold allowing optimal mechanical properties with minimal weight.*

Microscopically, woven and lamellar bone can be distinguished. Woven bone is the type formed initially in the embryo and during growth and is characterized by an irregular structure of loosely packed collagen fibrils. It is then replaced by the lamellar bone, so that it is practically no longer present in the adult skeleton, except in pathological conditions of rapid bone formation, such as in Paget's disease, fluorosis or fracture healing. In contrast, lamellar bone is the form present in the adult, both in cortical and cancellous bone. It is made of well ordered parallel collagen lamellae.

Paget's disease p. 71

> *Histologically bone formed during growth is of the woven type; in the adult it is lamellar.*

In cortical bone the tissue is mainly organized as osteons or Haversian systems, which represent its basic structural building blocks. These are tubes of up to 2 mm in length and 200 μm in diameter, made of concentric lamellae, between which the osteocytes are located. In the center is a canal containing the nutrient blood vessels. These anastomose with vessels from other osteons so that the various osteons are in communication with one another. The diameter of the osteon is always about 200 μm, regardless of species, the maximal distance of any part from the central vessel being no more than 100 μm, this being the distance nutrients are able to diffuse. Osteons are separated from one another by so-called cement lines.

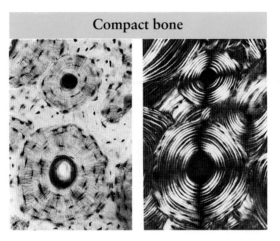

Compact bone

Fig. 1.1-1 Cross section of compact bone showing osteons with osteocytes (left), and – in polarized light – with collagen lamellae (right). (From Schenk, R.K. *et al.* (1993). Reproduced from Royce, P.M. and Steinmann, B. (eds.) (1993). *Connective Tissue and its Heritable Disorders. Molecular, Genetic, and Mineral Aspects*, pp. 85–101, with copyright permission from the author and John Wiley & Sons, Inc.)

The osteon is the basic unit of the Haversian bone of the cortex.

Remodeling of packets and BMUs p. 22

Osteoporosis p. 116

The trabeculae also consist of subunits which in this location are called 'packets'. They are separated, as are the osteons of the cortex, by cement lines. When they are on the surface and not yet terminated, they are called 'bone multicellular units' (BMUs). However, BMUs and packets are also found on the inner surface of the cortex, which therefore, looks very much like trabecular bone. These two locations, trabeculae and inner cortex, are those that are affected predominantly by osteoporosis.

Trabeculae generally possess no vessels and are therefore nourished from the surface. This explains why they cannot become much thicker than about 200–300 μm, twice the distance of 100 μm over which diffusion of nutrients is possible.

Fig. 1.1-2 Trabecular bone showing individual packets separated by cement lines. (Courtesy of Dr R.K. Schenk.)

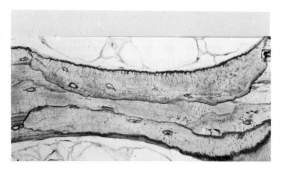

1.1.2. Composition of bone

Bone is made up essentially of mineral, organic matrix, cells and water.

Fig. 1.1-3 Composition of bone.

Composition of bone	
Mineral ~65%	Hydroxyapatite
Matrix ~35%	Collagen ~90% Other proteins Lipids
Cells	Osteoblasts Lining cells Osteocytes Osteoclasts
Water	

Mineral

The mineral amounts to about two-thirds of the total dry weight of bone. It is made of small crystals in the shape of needles, plates and rods located within and between the collagen fibrils. Chemically it is basically hydroxyapatite, $Ca_{10}(PO_4)_6(OH)_2$, although it is not pure but contains many other constituents, among others carbonate, citrate, magnesium, sodium, fluoride and strontium. These are either incorporated into the crystal lattice, or adsorbed onto the crystal surface. For this reason, the more general term calcium phosphate will be used in this book for bone mineral.

Deposition of bisphospho- nates in bone p. 58

Some substances, such as tetracyclines, polyphosphates and bisphos- phonates have a special affinity for calcium phosphate and hence for bone. They are deposited in preference on the mineral at sites of new bone formation. This 'bone seeking' property has been utilized in the case of tetracyclines in order to label newly formed bone, thus enabling the assessment of bone formation. Indeed, by administering tetracycline twice at a known time interval, the visualization of the fluorescent marker in bone biopsies enables the distance between the two lines of deposition to be measured and the amount of bone formed during this interval to be determined. The binding of polyphosphates and bisphos- phonates, when linked to ^{99m}Tc, is used in nuclear medicine to visualize hot spots of bone formation by scintigraphy. This technique is especially useful for detecting skeletal metastases and the osseous changes in Paget's disease. Lastly, the strong binding of bisphosphonates to bone mineral is fundamental to their pharmacological activity.

Paget's disease p. 70

The bone mineral is made essentially of impure calcium apatite. However, foreign substances such as tetracyclines, polyphosphates and bisphosphonates can also be incorporated with high affinity.

Organic matrix

The matrix amounts to about 35% of the dry weight of bone. It consists of 90% collagen, which is thus by far the most abundant bone protein. Its complex three-dimensional structure, comparable to that of a rope, gives bone its tensile strength.

The remainder of the bone matrix is made of various non-collagenous proteins, the role of which is not yet well understood. The most abun- dant ones are osteonectin, osteocalcin, also called bone gla-protein (BGP), osteopontin and bone sialoprotein.

Measurement of bone turnover p. 27

The urinary excretion and the plasma or serum levels of some of the components of the matrix are used clinically to assess bone turnover.

Bone matrix is made up of 90% collagen and about 10% of various non-collagenous proteins.

Bone cells

Osteoblasts

The osteoblasts, which derive from mesenchymal stem cells located in the bone marrow, are the cells that synthesize the bone matrix. They form an epithelial-like structure at the surface of the bone where they secrete uni-directionally the osseous organic matrix. In a second step, this matrix then calcifies extracellularly. As a consequence of the time lag between the formation of the matrix and its calcification, there is often a layer of unmineralized matrix under the osteoblasts. This diminishes in width when the rate of bone matrix formation decreases, but it widens when mineralization is delayed. This widening is most prominent when there is an arrest in mineralization, such as in osteomalacia. This is seen for example when large amounts of etidronate are given.

Etidronate-induced osteo-malacia
p. 148

Fig. 1.1-4   Lamellar bone formation with osteoblasts and osteoid seam. (Courtesy of Dr R.K. Schenk.)

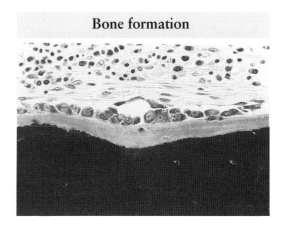

Bone formation

The modulation of bone formation is still poorly understood. It may occur at the level of the recruitment of new osteoblasts as well as through the alteration of osteoblast function. Although many hormones and cytokines influence osteoblasts *in vitro*, among them the insulin-like growth factors (IGFs), transforming growth factor β (TGFβ), acidic and basic fibroblast growth factors (FGFs), platelet-derived growth factor (PDGF), bone morphogenetic proteins (BMPs) and prostaglandins, their role *in vivo* is not yet clear.

One of the main aims of current research is to develop molecules that will increase bone formation. Up to now the only substances that are active in this direction, when given systemically, are fluoride, parathyroid hormone and certain cytokines such as prostaglandins and IGF-1. Of these only fluoride has been used therapeutically to date in clinical practice, namely in osteoporosis. Parathyroid hormone is under investigation. When locally administered in the proximity of bone in animals, various growth factors such as TGFβ, basic FGF, PDGF and BMPs induce bone formation at the site of injection. These as well as others, such as the IGFs, could prove useful in the future for such indications as improving fracture healing, filling osseous defects and possibly inducing

Fluoride in osteoporosis
p. 124

ridge augmentation in periodontology. Whether systemic administration will become possible is unknown. Effects on other organs are, however, likely to make this development difficult.

Corticosteroid-induced osteo-porosis
p. 118

In contrast, corticosteroids inhibit bone formation, explaining why chronic administration of these compounds leads both in animals and in humans to osteoporosis.

Bone formation	
Increase	**Decrease**
Systemic	
Fluoride	Corticosteroids
PTH	
Prostaglandins	
Cytokines	
Local	
BMPs FGFs	
TGFβ PDGF	
IGFs Prostaglandins	

Fig. 1.1-5 Possible physiological and pharmacological modulators of bone formation.

Bone is formed by the osteoblasts. Their modulation and therefore the modulation of bone formation are still little understood.

Lining cells

When the osteoblasts are not in the process of forming bone, they are flat and are called resting osteoblasts or lining cells. Active and resting osteoblasts form a membrane at the surface of the bone tissue, which may be important in constituting some kind of blood–bone barrier able to assure a characteristic osseous *milieu intérieur*.

Resting osteoblasts at the surface of the bone are called lining cells.

Osteocytes

At a certain moment the osteoblasts stop synthesizing matrix and become embedded within bone. They are then called osteocytes. Despite the fact that they are the most numerous cells in bone, their function is still poorly understood. They are located in lacunae and are intercon-nected by long cytoplasmic processes among themselves and with the osteoblasts. Gap junctions at the membrane contact sites make a func-tional syncytium, allowing bone to respond to stimuli over large areas. These cell processes are located within canaliculi, which contain, together with the lacunae, the so-called bone fluid. As the surface of these lacunae and canaliculi is very large, in humans about 1000 m^2, the bone fluid is in immediate contact with the mineral, with which it is in equi-librium. The osteocytes are thought to influence the composition of this bone fluid. Since the latter is also related to the extracellular fluid and therefore to blood, the osteocytes may play a role in the regulation of plasma minerals, especially calcium. Osteocytes are also well located for responding to mechanical stress and are thought today to play a key role in transducing mechanical loads into changes in bone formation and bone resorption.

Morphology of cell–cell connection p. 12

The role of the osteocytes is still little understood. They are probably involved in the homeostasis of bone fluid and con-sequently in the homeostasis of plasma calcium, and in the adaptation of bone in response to mechanical influences.

Osteoclasts

The fourth type of cell in bone is the osteoclast. It originates from a dif-ferent lineage to that of the other bone cells, namely from the hemo-poietic compartment, more precisely from the granulocyte–macrophage colony-forming unit (GM–CFU).

Fig. 1.1-6 Electron micrograph of an osteo-clast. (Reproduced from Schenk, R.K. (1974). *Verh. Dtsch. Ges. Pathol.*, 58, 72–83, with permission from the author and publisher.)

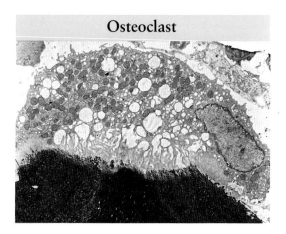

Osteoclast

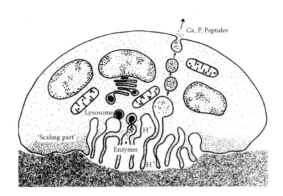

Fig. 1.1-7 Diagram of an osteoclast. N, nucleus. (Adapted from Schenk, R.K. (1974). *Verh. Dtsch. Ges. Pathol.*, 58, 72–83, with permission from the author and publisher.)

Remodeling
p. 20

Osteoclasts are usually large multinucleated cells that are situated either on the surface of the cortical or trabecular bone, often in depressions called Howship's lacunae, or within the cortical bone. There they are located at the tip of the remodeling units, burring the vascular canals in which the new osteons will be formed. Today some mononuclear precursors are also thought to be able to destroy bone and are thus called mononuclear osteoclasts.

The role of osteoclasts is to resorb bone. This is performed in a closed, sealed-off microenvironment located between the cell and the bone, called the clear zone, confined by the adherence of the cell rim to the bone. This attachment involves cell membrane receptors, called integrins, which recognize specific peptide sequences in the matrix. Covering this microenvironement is another specialized part of the cell membrane, called the ruffled border, which secretes two types of products, both leading to bone destruction. The first, the H^+ ions, which dissolve the bone mineral, originate from H_2CO_3 as a result of the action of carbonic anhydrase and are secreted by means of a proton ATPase. The second category includes various proteolytic enzymes, especially cathepsins and collagenases, which digest the matrix.

Current investigations are directed towards the development of specific inhibitors of these various proceses, with the aim to develop drugs that will decrease bone destruction.

Bone resorption can be modulated by altering two basic processes, namely the recruitment of new osteoclasts or the activity of mature osteoclasts. Both are influenced by a series of cytokines and hormones. Recent results indicate that both processes seem to be under the control of the cells of osteoblastic lineage, which synthesize some known factors, such as cytokines, and some as yet unknown factors, acting directly on the osteoclasts and their precursors.

Fig. 1.1-8 Regulation of bone resorption: role of the osteoblast.

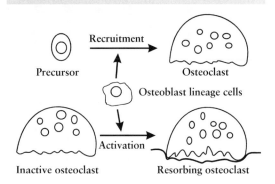

Osteoclast recruitment and activation

The three main hormones modulating bone resorption are parathyroid hormone (PTH), 1,25(OH)$_2$ vitamin D (calcitriol) and calcitonin, the first two increasing, the latter decreasing resorption. Furthermore, estrogens in women and testosterone in men inhibit bone resorption, in part at least by decreasing the production of interleukin (IL)-6. Menopause and ovariectomy, as well as orchidectomy, induce a dramatic increase in bone resorption, mediated apparently by an increase in IL-6. Among the most important cytokines that can increase bone resorption, at least *in vitro*, and are possibly involved in this process *in vivo*, are the interleukins 1, 3, 6 and 11 (IL-1, IL-3, IL-6, IL-11), tumor necrosis factor α and β (TNFα, TNFβ), macrophage colony-stimulating factor

Calcium homeostasis p. 24

Fig. 1.1-9 Possible modulators of bone resorption.

Bone resorption

Increase		Decrease
Systemic		
PTH		Calcitonin
PTHrP		Estrogen
Calcitriol		
Thyroxin		
Local		
IL-1		
IL-6	TNFα	TGFβ
IL-11	TNFβ	IFNγ
FGFs	TGFβ	IL-4
Prostaglandins	M-CSF	

(M-CSF), granulocyte–macrophage colony-stimulating factor (GM-CSF), stem cell factor (SCF) and prostaglandins. Interferon γ (IFNγ), TGFβ, IL-4 and IL-13 on the other hand, decrease bone resorption. Some of these cytokines are produced by the cells of osteoblastic lineage and are therefore possibly involved in the osteoblast–osteoclast axis.

> *Bone resorption is performed by the osteoclast. Its recruitment and activity is under the modulation of a series of hormones and cytokines and under the control of the cells of osteoblastic lineage.*

1.1.3. Modeling and remodeling

Bone is continuously being turned over by the two processes of modeling and remodeling. In the former, which takes place principally in the child, new bone is formed at a location different from the one destroyed. This therefore results in a change in the shape of the skeleton. It allows not only the development of a normal architecture during growth, but also the modulation of this architecture in the adult when the mechanical conditions change. Furthermore it is the cause of the increase in size of the vertebrae during life. In remodeling, which is the main process in the adult, the two processes occur in the same place, so that no change occurs in the shape of the bone. Both modeling and remodeling, however, result in the replacement of old bone by new bone. This allows the maintenance of the mechanical integrity of the skeleton, which is illustrated by the fact that in diseases where bone resorption is impaired, such as in osteopetrosis, bone becomes fragile and fractures occur. The turnover also allows the bone to play its role as an ion bank.

Biomechanical adaptation p. 26

Calcium homeostasis p. 25

The remodeling rate is between 2% and 10% of the skeletal mass per year. It is increased by parathyroid hormone, thyroxin, growth hormone and 1,25(OH)$_2$ vitamin D, decreased by calcitonin, estrogen and glucocorticosteroids. It is also stimulated by microfractures and modulated by the mechanical conditions. The cancellous bone, which represents about 20% of the skeletal mass, makes up 80% of the turnover, while the cortex, which represents 80% of the bone, makes up only 20% of the turnover. This explains why osteoporosis, which is the result of an abnormal turnover, is seen first and mainly in cancellous bone.

Osteoporosis p. 116

> *Bone is continuously turned over by modeling and remodeling, the rates of which are under hormonal influence. Cancellous bone accounts for 80% of the turnover, although it represents only 20% of the skeleton.*

Fig. 1.1-10 Cortical bone remodeling. Osteoclasts located at the tip of the cone erode a canal within the bone. Osteoblasts present on the lateral walls will refill it and form the osteon. (From Schenk, R.K. *et al.* (1993). Reproduced from Royce, P.M. and Steinman, B. (eds.) *Connective Tissue and its Heritable Disorders. Molecular, Genetic, and Mineral Aspects*, pp. 85–101, with copyright permission from the author and John Wiley & Sons, Inc.)

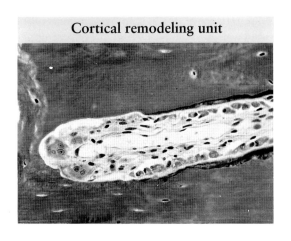

Cortical remodeling unit

Fig. 1.1-11 Cancellous bone remodeling. The process starts with erosion of the surface by osteoclasts, followed by refilling of the cavity by osteoblasts. (From Schenk, R.K. *et al.* (1993). Reproduced from Royce, P.M. and Steinman, B. (eds.) *Connective Tissue and its Heritable Disorders. Molecular, Genetic, and Mineral Aspects*, pp. 85–101, with copyright permission from the author and John Wiley & Sons, Inc.)

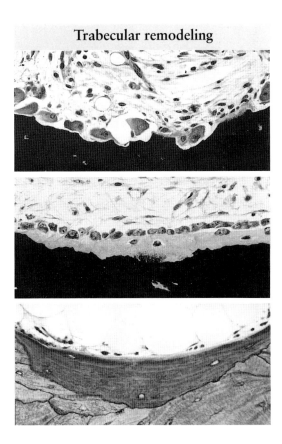

Trabecular remodeling

BMUs
BSUs
p. 12
The morphological dynamic substrate of turnover is the 'bone multi- ←
cellular unit' (BMU), also called 'bone remodeling unit' (BRU). The morphological entity formed when the process is terminated is called the
'bone structural unit' (BSU) which corresponds to the packet in cancellous bone, and to the osteon in cortical bone. Both in the cortex and in ←
the trabeculae, the process of remodeling starts in the same way by bone
being eroded by osteoclasts. In a second step, the resorption sites are
refilled by the osteoblasts. The linear resorption rate of osteoclasts is
about 50 µm per day. The formation is slower, about 1 µm per day for
lamellar, more for woven bone. The time required for the destruction
and reconstruction of a complete BSU is between 3 and 5 months.

The basic dynamic unit of bone remodeling is the BMU.

Normally the amount of bone formed equals the amount destroyed, ←
so that the balance is zero. The mechanism underlying this 'coupling'
between the resorption and the formation processes is still unknown and
the subject of intensive investigation. Its elucidation may explain the
Osteoporosis
p. 119
cause of osteoporosis, in which more bone is being destroyed than
formed, resulting in a negative balance. This imbalance is seen for example after the menopause or during immobilization.

**In the steady state, the amount of bone formed in the remodeling
process equals the amount destroyed. If more bone is destroyed
than formed, bone loss occurs and osteoporosis may develop.**

A special situation arises in periods where turnover rates change, for
example after the administration of an inhibitor of bone resorption.
Since there is a time interval between the beginning of the inhibition of
the resorption process and the start of the secondary decrease in formation, a transient net gain of bone will occur whenever the turnover rate
decreases. This time interval explains why after the administration of an
Turnover
markers
p. 73
inhibitor of bone resorption, such as a bisphosphonate, markers of bone
resorption such as urinary hydroxyproline decrease sooner than markers
of bone formation such as alkaline phosphatase. The volume of bone
gained in this way, sometimes called the remodeling space, may account
for up to a total of 2%, more for trabecular bone volume, or when the
turnover is rapid, less for the cortex. Furthermore, after inhibition of
turnover, some calcium will still be taken up by the not yet completely
mineralized matrix, accounting for another 1–2% increase of calcium.
Thus a total elevation of 3–4% in skeletal calcium, and therefore of bone
mineral density, may occur, possibly more if turnover is higher. Such an
increase in bone mass is seen with various inhibitors of bone resorption

such as estrogens, calcitonin and bisphosphonates. It is, however, not a true durable augmentation in bone mass, but a transient one that will be reversed if the inhibition is stopped, a fact that has often been neglected in the literature. In contrast, the gain in bone mass may remain if bone turnover is maintained at the lower level.

Bisphos-
phonates in
osteoporosis
pp. 126–127

→ Fig. 1.1-12 Influence of changes in turnover on calcium balance.

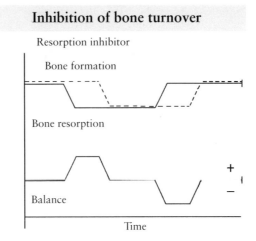

Inhibition of bone turnover

When turnover rate is decreased, a transient increase of bone mass occurs, which, however, is reversed as soon as turnover normalizes again.

1.1.4. Calcium homeostasis

Calcium concentration in plasma is around 10 mg per 100 ml. About 40% of this is bound to proteins and 10% to ultrafilterable ions, so that approximately half only is ionized. The level of ionized plasma calcium and not of total calcium is the fraction that is tightly controlled throughout the animal world. This has led some authors to call ionized calcium one of nature's physiological constants. This constancy is explained by the importance of extracellular calcium for many biological processes. Nevertheless, for clinical purposes, and as long as there is no disturbance in plasma proteins and plasma pH, measurement of total calcium is usually sufficient. In some conditions, however, such as in tumor bone disease, plasma proteins are disturbed to such an extent that a correction is necessary.

Correction
for plasma
proteins
p. 90

Plasma ionized calcium, and not total calcium, is the fraction that is tightly controlled.

The level of ionized calcium, and therefore of plasma calcium, is set by ← the interaction of the three target organs, intestine, bone and kidney. Calcemia will depend upon the fluxes between extracellular fluid and therefore blood, and these three organs.

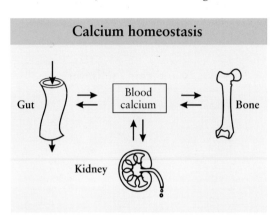

Fig. 1.1-13   Calcium homeostasis in the body.

Bone resorption p. 19
The fluxes are controlled mainly by three hormones, parathyroid hor- ← mone (PTH), the vitamin D metabolite $1,25(OH)_2$ vitamin D (calcitriol) and possibly calcitonin, although the last has not yet been proven to act physiologically. All three are directly regulated by calcemia through a feed-back mechanism.

Blood calcium is regulated mainly by the three hormones parathyroid hormone, $1,25(OH)_2$ vitamin D and possibly calcitonin.

Of the three hormones, the most important is parathyroid hormone, ← which increases calcemia by action on all three target organs. Thus it increases bone resorption, increases the intestinal absorption of calcium, although indirectly through an elevation of $1,25(OH)_2$ vitamin D, and increases renal tubular reabsorption of calcium. Since the production of parathyroid hormone is inversely related to calcemia and is rapidly modulated, this hormone provides an excellent rapidly working negative feed-back mechanism.

The hormone $1,25(OH)_2$ vitamin D increases intestinal calcium absorption and bone resorption. Since its production is stimulated by low plasma calcium, it also provides a regulatory feed-back mechanism.

However, in contrast to parathyroid hormone, which is modulated and acts within minutes, 1,25(OH)$_2$ vitamin D requires hours to days. Vitamin D metabolites are also required for normal mineralization of bone.

Finally, calcitonin inhibits bone destruction. This property is used therapeutically in diseases with increased bone resorption, such as Paget's disease and osteoporosis. Since its production is rapidly modulated by calcemia through positive feed-back, this hormone could also theoretically provide good feed-back regulation. Its relevance in humans for calcium homeostasis is, however, not yet established.

Calcitonin in Paget's disease p. 72
Calcitonin in osteoporosis p. 123

Fig. 1.1-14 Role of parathyroid hormone, 1,25(OH)$_2$ vitamin D and calcitonin in calcium homeostasis.

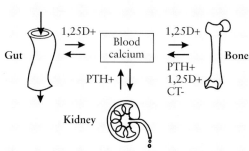

Hormones and calcium homeostasis

Parathyroid hormone, 1,25(OH)$_2$ vitamin D and calcitonin are all regulated by calcemia, providing an excellent homeostatic feed-back mechanism for maintaining plasma calcium homeostasis.

Thus the three target organs, intestine, kidney and bone, are intimately linked with respect to calcium homeostasis. Consequently, a disturbance in one of these organs will affect the others. Since 99% of the body calcium is located in the skeleton, this will act as a reserve of the ion. In the case of calcium shortage, the homeostatic mechanisms will work to the detriment of the bone in order to maintain calcemia, which seems to have absolute priority. It is not yet clear what the daily intake of calcium should be for humans. It is thought today that 1g is necessary in adult life, somewhat more in adolescents, and 1.5 g in the elderly as well as during pregnancy and lactation. If this is true, a large part of the population would be chronically calcium deficient, since its daily intake is usually only about 0.5 g. It is interesting that in the animal kingdom, humans have by far the lowest calcium intake by body weight. Calcium

Calcium in osteoporosis p. 118 p. 123

deficiency may possibly explain in part the bone loss during the second part of life, since calcium absorption decreases in the elderly, who can have a vitamin D deficiency or a disturbance in its metabolism and action. A decrease in calcium absorption due to malabsorption or to a deficiency in calcium intake, or a loss in the urine such as in renal hypercalciuria, may also induce bone loss.

1.1.5. Bone as an organ

In addition to these homeostatic mechanisms at the service of plasma calcium, other mechanisms exist which allow bone to maintain its own integrity. First microcracks, which occur constantly during life, stimulate bone remodeling. Then, the strains induced by outside mechanical influences most probably play a primordial role in both modeling and remodeling. This system also has a feed-back loop, since a loss of bone will increase the strains induced, leading to increased bone formation and/or decreased bone resorption, and therefore a subsequent increase in bone mass. These mechanisms also allow bone to adapt its structure to function and to fulfil its mechanical role optimally. They explain why the trabeculae of cancellous bone are oriented along the prevailing lines of pressure and traction and why they change if these are altered, for example after an orthopedic operation that alters the axis, or locally after destruction of individual trabeculae (*see* Fig. 1.1-15).

On the other hand, a disturbance in mechanical function, such as in immobilization, leads to rapid and massive bone loss, as seen in plaster-immobilized limbs or after paralysis. The magnitude of the bone loss can be such as to disturb calcium homeostasis and lead to hypercalciuria and even hypercalcemia. Some bone loss also occurs during weightlessness in astronauts. Therefore, one of the rules in osteoporotic patients is to avoid immobilization. The cellular mechanisms underlying these events are yet little understood but are likely to involve the osteocytes and local cytokines.

Mechanical forces influence bone turnover and allow the skeleton to maintain an optimal structure to fulfil its mechanical function. Immobilization induces bone loss.

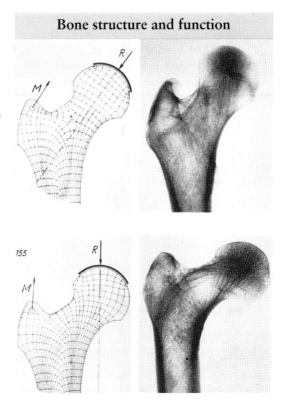

Fig. 1.1-15 Adaptation of bone structure to mechanical function along lines of pressure and tension.
M, muscle pull; R, down direction of load.
(Adapted from Pauwels, F. (1960). *Z. Anat. Entwickl. Gesch.*, **121**, 478–515, with permission from the publisher).

→ ## 1.1.6. Assessment of bone turnover

Bone turnover can be assessed *in vivo*, although only indirectly. For bone formation the measurements most commonly used are serum alkaline phosphatase, preferentially the bone isoenzyme, and serum osteocalcin. Alkaline phosphatase is produced by the osteoblasts during bone formation. Osteocalcin is specific to bone and is liberated during the formation of matrix by the osteoblasts. Its level in serum is a good index for bone formation, except, for unknown reasons, in Paget's disease. More recently the appearance of certain propeptides liberated during collagen synthesis has been used.

Markers in Paget's disease p. 71

→ Bone resorption is evaluated by measuring the urinary excretion of bone collagen breakdown products such as hydroxyproline, pyridinoline crosslinks and certain collagen fragments. Collagen contains 10% hydroxyproline. When bone is destroyed, some of this amino acid is excreted in the urine, so that urinary hydroxyproline can be used as an index of bone destruction. However, since urinary hydroxyproline can also originate from non-osseous collagen, and since some of the amino acid is metabolized, this index is not ideal by far. Furthermore it is also absorbed from dietary collagen, so that the measurements must be performed under a collagen-free diet. The procedure can be simplified by measuring the hydroxyproline/creatinine ratio of the first 2-h morning fasting urine specimen obtained after the urine of the night is voided, and with no intake of collagen the evening before.

Better markers of bone resorption are the pyridinoline crosslinks present in collagen. These are formed by the linkage of two collagen molecules to form pyridinoline and deoxypyridinoline. Of the two, only the latter is specific to bone. Nevertheless, for an unknown reason, both measurements seem to give similar results, so that often both are measured together. No dietary precautions are necessary. Until recently this determination was performed only in specialized laboratories by means of high-performance liquid chromatography, but the development of immunoassays makes it now more widely available. Very recently antibodies have been developed against pyridinoline-containing peptides appearing in the urine which appear to give excellent results.

Lastly, a negative calcium balance may be visualized sometimes by measuring the morning fasting urinary calcium/creatinine ratio.

Bone formation is assessed by measuring serum alkaline phosphatase and osteocalcin, bone resorption by measuring urinary hydroxyproline and pyridinoline crosslinks or peptides containing these crosslinks.

Recommended selected reading

Books

Coe, F.L. and Favus, M.J. (eds.) (1992). *Disorders of Bone and Mineral Metabolism*. (New York, Raven Press)

Favus, M.J. (ed.) (1993). *Primer on the Metabolic Bone Diseases and Disorders of Mineral Metabolism*, 2nd edn. (New York, Raven Press)

Mundy, G.R. (1995). Bone remodeling and its disorders. (London: Martin Dunitz)

Mundy, G.R. and Martin, T.J. (eds.) (1993). *Physiology and Pharmacology of Bone. Handbook of Experimental Pharmacology*, vol. 107. (Berlin, Heidelberg, New York: Springer-Verlag)

Noda, M. (ed.) (1993). *Cellular and Molecular Biology of Bone*. (San Diego: Academic Press)

Reviews

Morphology

Eriksen, E.F., Vesterby, A., Kassem, M., Melsen, F. and Mosekilde, L. (1993). Bone remodeling and bone structure. In Mundy, G.R. and Martin, T.J. (eds.) *Physiology and Pharmacology of Bone. Handbook of Experimental Pharmacology*, vol. 107, pp. 67–109. (Berlin, Heidelberg, New York: Springer-Verlag)

Parfitt, A.M. (1992). The physiologic and pathogenetic significance of bone histomorphometric data. In Coe, F.L. and Favus, M.J. (eds.) *Disorders of Bone and Mineral Metabolism*, pp. 475–89. (New York: Raven Press)

Recker, R.R. (1992). Embryology, anatomy, and microstructure of bone. In Coe, F.L. and Favus, M.J. (eds.) *Disorders of Bone and Mineral Metabolism*. pp. 219–40. (New York: Raven Press)

Schenk, R.K., Felix, R. and Hofstetter, W. (1993). Morphology of connective tissue: bone. In Royce, P.M. and Steinmann, B. (eds.) *Connective Tissue and Its Heritable Disorders. Molecular, Genetic, and Medical Aspects*, pp. 85–101. (New York: Wiley-Liss)

Chemistry

Delmas, P.D. and Malaval, L. (1993). The proteins of bone. In Mundy, G.R. and Martin, T.J. (eds.) *Physiology and Pharmacology of Bone. Handbook of Experimental Pharmacology*, vol. 107, pp. 673–724. (Berlin, Heidelberg, New York: Springer-Verlag)

Gehron Robey, P., Bianco, P. and Termine, J.D. (1992). The cellular biology and molecular biochemistry of bone formation. In Coe, F.L. and Favus, M.J. (eds.) *Disorders of Bone and Mineral Metabolism*, pp. 241–63. (New York: Raven Press, Ltd)

Young M.F., Ibaraki K., Kerr J.M. and Heegard A.-M. (1993). Molecular and cellular biology of the major noncollagenous proteins in bone. In Noda M. (ed.) *Cellular and Molecular Biology of Bone*, pp. 191–234. (San Diego: Academic Press)

Cells

Aarden, E.M., Burger, E.H. and Nijweide, P.J. (1994). Function of osteocytes in bone. *J. Cell. Biochem.*, **55**, 287–99

Aubin, J.E., Turksen, K. and Heersche, J.N.M. (1993). Osteoblastic cell lineage. In Noda, M. (ed.) *Cellular and Molecular Biology of Bone*, pp. 1–45. (San Diego: Academic Press)

Baron, R., Chakraborty, M., Chatterjee, D., Horne, W., Lomri, A. and Ravesloot, J.-H. (1993). Biology of the osteoclast. In Mundy, G.R. and Martin, T.J. (eds.) *Physiology and Pharmacology of Bone. Handbook of Experimental Pharmacology*, vol. 107, pp. 111–47. (Berlin, Heidelberg, New York: Springer-Verlag)

Martin, T.J., Findlay, D.M., Heath, J.K. and Ng, K.W. (1993). Osteoblast: differentiation and function. In Mundy, G.R. and Martin, T.J. (eds.) *Physiology and Pharmacology of Bone. Handbook of Experimental Pharmacology*, vol. 107, pp. 149–83. (Berlin, Heidelberg, New York: Springer-Verlag)

Suda, T., Takahashi, N. and Martin, T.J. (1992). Modulation of osteoclast differentiation. *Endocr. Rev.*, **13**, 66–80

Bone formation and resorption

Canalis, E., McCarthy, T.L. and Centrella, M. (1993). Factors that regulate bone formation. In Mundy, G.R. and Martin, T.J. (eds.) *Physiology and Pharmacology of Bone. Handbook of Experimental Pharmacology*, vol. 107, pp. 249–66. (Berlin, Heidelberg, New York: Springer-Verlag)

Centrella, M., McCarthy, T.L. and Canalis, E. (1992). Growth factors and cytokines. In Hall, B.K. (ed.) *Bone*, vol. 4, *Bone Metabolism and Mineralization*, pp. 47–72. (Boca Raton, Ann Arbor, London: CRC Press)

Dempster, D.W. (1992). Bone remodeling. In Coe, F.L. and Favus, M.J. (eds.) *Disorders of Bone and Mineral Metabolism*, pp. 355–80. (New York: Raven Press)

Gowen, M. (1994) Cytokines and cellular interactions in the control of bone remodelling. In Heersche, J.N.M. and Kanis, J.A. (eds.) *Bone and Mineral Research*, pp. 77–114. (Amsterdam, London, New York, Tokyo: Elsevier)

Manolagas, S.C. and Jilka, R.L. (1995). Bone marrow, cytokines, and bone remodeling. *N. Engl. J. Med.*, **332**, 305–11

Mohan, S. and Baylink, D.J. (1991). Bone growth factors. *Clin. Orthop.*, **263**, 30–48

Mundy, G.R. (1993). Cytokines of bone. In Mundy, G.R. and Martin, T.J. (eds.) *Physiology and Pharmacology of Bone. Handbook of Experimental Pharmacology*, vol. 107, pp. 215–47. (Berlin, Heidelberg, New York: Springer-Verlag)

Mundy, G.R. (1993). Hormonal factors which regulate bone resorption. In Mundy, G.R. and Martin, T.J. (eds.) *Physiology and Pharmacology of Bone. Handbook of Experimental Pharmacology*, vol. 107, pp. 185–214. (Berlin, Heidelberg, New York: Springer-Verlag)

Raisz, L.G. (1992). Mechanisms and regulation of bone resorption by osteoclastic cells. In Coe, F.L. and Favus, M.J. (eds.) *Disorders of Bone and Mineral Metabolism*, pp. 287–311. (New York: Raven Press)

Calcium homeostasis

Bushinsky, D.A. and Krieger, N.S. (1992). Integration of calcium metabolism in the adult. In Coe, F.L. and Favus, M.J. (eds.) *Disorders of Bone and Mineral Metabolism*, pp. 417–32. (New York: Raven Press)

Eisman, J.A. (1993). Vitamin D metabolism. In Mundy, G.R. and Martin, T.J. (eds.) *Physiology and Pharmacology of Bone. Handbook of Experimental Pharmacology*, vol. 107, pp. 333–75. (Berlin, Heidelberg, New York: Springer-Verlag)

Mundy, G.R. (1990). General concepts of calcium homeostasis. – Calcium homeostasis – role of the gut, kidney and bone. – Hormonal factors which influence calcium homeostasis. In Mundy, G.R. (ed.) *Calcium Homeostasis: Hypercalcemia and Hypocalcemia*, 2nd edn, pp. 1–54. (London: Martin Dunitz)

Parfitt, A.M. (1993). Calcium homeostasis. In Mundy, G.R. and Martin, T.J. (eds.) *Physiology and Pharmacology of Bone. Handbook of Experimental Pharmacology*, vol. 107, pp. 1–65. (Berlin, Heidelberg, New York: Springer-Verlag)

Wendelaar Bonga, S.E. and Pang, P.K.T. (1991). Control of calcium regulating hormones in the vertebrates: parathyroid hormone, calcitonin, prolactin, and stanniocalcin. *Int. Rev. Cytol.*, **128**, 139–213

2. Bisphosphonates – preclinical

2.1. BACKGROUND TO THE PHARMACOLOGICAL DEVELOPMENT

Our knowledge of the biological characteristics of bisphosphonates dates from more than 25 years ago, the first report having appeared in 1968. The concept was derived from earlier studies in our laboratory on inorganic pyrophosphate. We had found that plasma and urine contained compounds inhibiting calcium phosphate precipitation, and that part of this inhibitory activity was due to inorganic pyrophosphate, a substance that had not been described previously in these media.

Fig. 2.1-1 Chemical structure of inorganic pyrophosphate.

Pyrophosphate

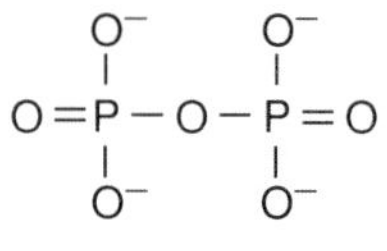

Pyrophosphate is the simplest of the condensed phosphates, compounds which have been used extensively in industry because of their property of inhibiting the precipitation of calcium carbonate. Their main applications were as antiscaling additives in washing powders, water and oil brines to prevent deposition of calcium carbonate scale.

31

Polyphosphates as antiscaling agents

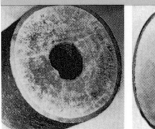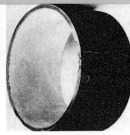

Fig. 2.1-2   Effect of polyphosphates on the deposition of calcium carbonate in a water pipe. (Adapted from Rudy, H. (1960). *Altes und Neues über kondensierte Phosphate*. (Ludwigshafen am Rhein: J.A. Benckiser, GmbH). Reproduced with permission from the publisher.)

Inorganic pyrophosphate, a compound used industrially for its property of inhibiting calcium carbonate, is present in biological fluids.

We then found that pyrophosphate binds very avidly to calcium phosphate and impairs not only the formation of calcium phosphate crystals *in vitro*, but also their dissolution. Pyrophosphate was then shown to inhibit calcification, also *in vivo*. Various types of ectopic calcification were efficiently prevented by the parenteral but not the oral administration of the compound. In contrast, no effect was found on bone resorption. This was explained by the possible hydrolysis of pyrophosphate when given orally and at the sites of bone destruction. These results led us to propose that pyrophosphate might be a physiological regulator of calcification and perhaps also of decalcification *in vivo*, its local concentration being determined by the pyrophosphatase activity of local phosphatases.

Inorganic pyrophosphate inhibits both the formation and the dissolution of calcium phosphate in vitro. In vivo it prevents ectopic calcification. It might be a regulator of mineral deposition and dissolution in the organism.

Because of its failure to act when given orally as a result of its rapid hydrolysis, pyrophosphate found a therapeutic use only in two indications. In view of its strong affinity for calcium phosphate and therefore for bone mineral, it is used, when linked to ^{99m}Tc, in skeletal scintigraphy. Furthermore, it is now the main antitartar agent in toothpastes world-wide.

Pyrophosphate is used in scintigraphy and as an antitartar agent in toothpastes.

This restricted use prompted us to search for analogs which would display similar physicochemical activity, but which would resist enzymatic hydrolysis and would therefore not be broken down metabolically. We found that the bisphosphonates fulfilled these conditions. In the last 30 years our group has worked, in collaboration with various pharmaceutical companies, on the development of the bisphosphonates and the elucidation of their mode of action.

Recommended selected reading

Reviews

Fleisch, H. and Russell, R.G.G. (1970). Pyrophosphate and polyphosphate. In *Encyclopaedia (Int.) of Pharmacology and Therapeutics*, Section 51. *Pharmacology of the Endocrine System and Related Drugs*, pp. 61–100. (Oxford, New York: Pergamon Press)

Original articles

Fleisch, H. and Bisaz, S. (1962). Isolation from urine of pyrophosphate, a calcification inhibitor. *Am. J. Physiol.*, **203**, 671–5

Fleisch, H. and Neuman, W.F. (1961). Mechanisms of calcification: role of collagen, polyphosphates and phosphatase. *Am. J. Physiol.*, **200**, 1296–300

Fleisch, H., Russell, R.G.G., Bisaz, S., Casey, P.A. and Mühlbauer, R.C. (1968). The influence of pyrophosphate analogues (diphosphonates) on the precipitation and dissolution of calcium phosphate *in vitro* and *in vivo*. *Calcif. Tissue Res.*, **2** (Suppl.), 10–10A

Fleisch, H., Russell, R.G.G. and Straumann, F. (1966). Effect of pyrophosphate on hydroxyapatite and its implications in calcium homeostasis. *Nature (London)*, **212**, 901–3

Russell, R.G.G., Bisaz, S., Donath, A., Morgan, D.B. and Fleisch, H. (1971). Inorganic pyrophosphate in plasma in normal persons and in patients with hypophosphatasia, osteogenesis imperfecta and other disorders of bone. *J. Clin. Invest.*, **50**, 961–9

Schibler, D., Russell, R.G.G. and Fleisch, H. (1968). Inhibition by pyrophosphate and polyphosphate of aortic calcification induced by vitamin D_3 in rats. *Clin. Sci.*, **35**, 363–72

2.2. Chemistry

Bisphosphonates, formerly called diphosphonates in error, are compounds characterized by two C-P bonds. If the two bonds are located on the same carbon atom, resulting in a P-C-P structure, the compounds are called geminal bisphosphonates. They are therefore analogs of pyrophosphate that contain a carbon instead of an oxygen atom. For the sake of simplicity, and since so far only P-C-P bisphosphonates have been found to exert strong activity on the skeleton, the geminal bisphosphonates will simply be called bisphosphonates in this book. This simplification is usually also made in the literature.

Chemical structure

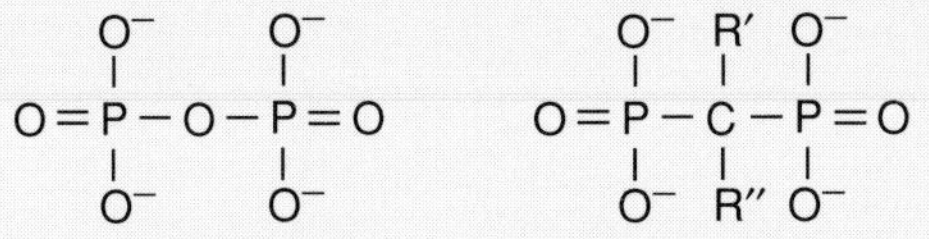

$$O = \overset{\overset{\textstyle O^-}{|}}{P} - O - \overset{\overset{\textstyle O^-}{|}}{\underset{\underset{\textstyle O^-}{|}}{P}} = O$$

Pyrophosphate

$$O = \overset{\overset{\textstyle O^-}{|}}{\underset{\underset{\textstyle O^-}{|}}{P}} - \overset{\overset{\textstyle R'}{|}}{\underset{\underset{\textstyle R''}{|}}{C}} - \overset{\overset{\textstyle O^-}{|}}{\underset{\underset{\textstyle O^-}{|}}{P}} = O$$

Geminal bisphosphonate

Fig. 2.2-1 Chemical structure of pyrophosphate and bisphosphonates.

Geminal bisphosphonates, called simply bisphosphonates in this book, are synthetic compounds characterized by P-C-P bonds.

The P-C-P structure allows a great number of possible variations, either by changing the two lateral chains on the carbon atom, or by esterifying the phosphate groups. The following bisphosphonates, in order of their chronological description, have been investigated in humans with respect to their effect on bone. Alendronate, clodronate, etidronate, pamidronate and tiludronate are commercially available in some countries (*see* Fig. 2.2-2)

Each bisphosphonate has its own physicochemical and biological characteristics. This variability in effect makes it impossible to extrapolate with certainty from data for one compound to others, so that each compound has to be considered on its own, with respect to both its use and its toxicology.

Many bisphosphonates have been investigated. Each has its own characteristic profile of activity.

Chemical structure pp. 35–36

Commercial index pp. 157–170

Bisphosphonates used in humans

(4-Amino-1-hydroxybutylidene)-bis-phosphonate

alendronate*

Gentili; Merck Sharp & Dohme

[(Cycloheptylamino)-methylene]bis-phosphonate

cimadronate

Yamanouchi

(Dichloromethylene)-bis-phosphonate

clodronate*

Astra; Boehringer Mannheim; Gentili; Leiras; Rhône-Poulenc Rorer

[1-Hydroxy-3-(1-pyrrolidinyl)-propylidene]bis-phosphonate

EB-1053

Leo

(1-Hydroxyethylidene)-bis-phosphonate

etidronate*

Gentili; Procter & Gamble

[1-Hydroxy-3-(methylpentylamino)propylidene]bis-phosphonate

ibandronate

Boehringer Mannheim

(6-Amino-1-hydroxyhexy-lidene)bis-phosphonate

neridronate

Gentili

[3-(Dimethylamino)-1-hydroxy-propylidene]bis-phosphonate

olpadronate

Gador

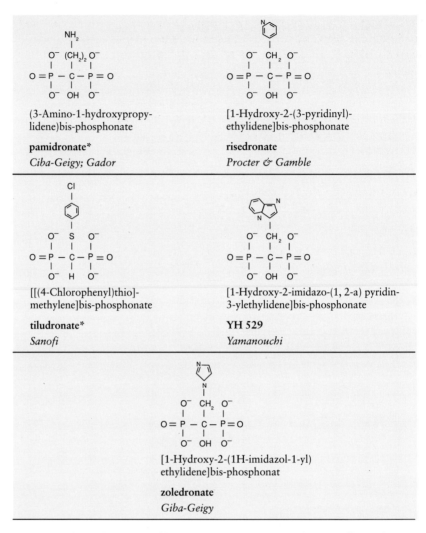

Fig. 2.2-2 Chemical structure of bisphosphonates investigated for their effect on bone in humans. *Commercially available.

The P-C-P bonds of the bisphosphonates are stable to heat and most chemical reagents, and completely resistant to enzymatic hydrolysis, but can be hydrolyzed in solution by ultraviolet light. These compounds have a strong affinity for metal ions, with which they can form both soluble and insoluble complexes and aggregates, depending on the pH of the ← solution and the metal present. This can occur *in vivo* when large amounts are infused rapidly, so that great care has to be taken when

Adverse events
p. 146

these compounds are given intravenously. Some uncertainty still exists as to the state of bisphosphonates when in solution. In plasma they are only partially ultrafilterable, which is of importance when renal clearance is calculated.

Ultrafilterability
p. 58

Clearance
p. 60

Bisphosphonates are resistant to chemical and enzymatic hydrolysis. They can form insoluble complexes.

Recommended selected reading

Review

Francis, M.D. and Martodam, R.R. (1983). Chemical, biochemical, and medicinal properties of the diphosphonates. In: Hilderbrand, R.L. (ed.) *The Role of Phosphonates in Living Systems*, pp. 55–96. (Boca Raton, Florida: CRC Press)

2.3. ACTIONS

2.3.1. Physicochemical effects

The physicochemical effects of many of the bisphosphonates are very similar to those of pyrophosphate. Thus, they inhibit the formation, delay the aggregation, and also slow down the dissolution of calcium phosphate crystals. All these effects are related to the marked affinity of these compounds for solid-phase calcium phosphate, on the surface of which they bind strongly. This effect is of great importance, since it is the basis for the use of these compounds as skeletal markers in nuclear medicine and the basis of their action on bone resorption when used as drugs.

Effects on calcium phosphate
• Bind strongly to crystals
• Inhibit crystal formation
• Inhibit crystal aggregation
• Inhibit crystal dissolution

Fig. 2.3-1 Physico-chemical effects of bisphosphonates on calcium phosphate.

Bisphosphonates also inhibit the formation and the aggregation of calcium oxalate crystals.

Bisphosphonates bind avidly to calcium phosphate crystals and inhibit their growth, aggregation and dissolution. The affinity for bone mineral is the basis for their use as skeletal markers and as inhibitors of bone resorption.

2.3.2. Biological effects

Inhibition of bone resorption

The main effect of the pharmacologically active bisphosphonates is to inhibit bone resorption. Indeed these compounds proved to be extremely powerful inhibitors of resorption when tested in a variety of conditions, both *in vitro* and *in vivo*.

In vitro

Bisphosphonates block bone resorption induced by various means in cell and organ culture. In the former, they inhibit the formation of pits by isolated osteoclasts cultured on mineralized substrata. In organ culture they decrease the destruction of bone in embryonic long bones and in neonatal calvaria. This inhibition is present whether resorption is stimulated or not. Up to now, all the stimulators of bone resorption, such as parathyroid hormone, 1, 25 $(OH)_2$ vitamin D and prostaglandins, as well as the products of tumor cells, have been inhibited in their effects.

Fig. 2.3-2 Effect of bisphosphonates on resorption of rat calvaria in culture, assayed by ^{45}Ca release. Open circles, etidronate; closed circles, clodronate. (Adapted from Reynolds, J.J. et al. (1972). Reproduced from *Calcified Tissue Res.*, **10**, 302–13, with copyright permission from the author and Springer-Verlag, Heidelberg.)

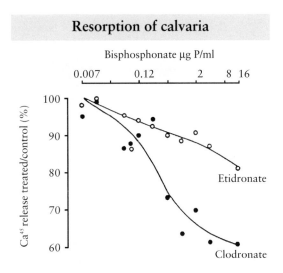

Until recently the correlation between the results obtained in calvaria *in vitro* and those obtained *in vivo* was rather poor. Recently, however, a study performed with nine compounds varying in their activity by 5–6 orders of magnitude showed a satisfactory correlation using the 4–7 day-old mouse calvaria assay.

Fig. 2.3-3 Inhibitory activity of various bisphosphonates *in vitro* in mouse calvariae and *in vivo* in the TPTX rat. (Adapted from Green, J.R. et al. (1994) with permission from the author and publisher.)

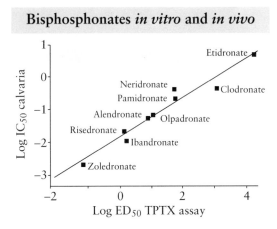

Bisphosphonates inhibit bone resorption in cell and organ culture.

Intact animals

In growing rats, bisphosphonates can block the degradation of both primary and secondary trabeculae, thus arresting the modeling and remodeling of the metaphysis. The latter therefore becomes club-shaped and radiologically more dense than normal, leading to a picture similar to that seen in congenital osteopetrotic animals. This effect is currently used as a model to estimate the potency of new compounds.

Inhibition of bone resorption

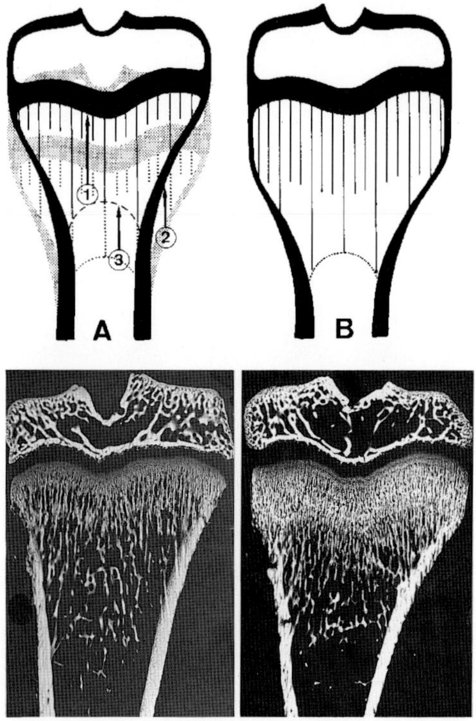

Fig 2.3-4 Inhibition of metaphyseal modeling and remodeling by a bisphosphonate in the growing rat. *Upper panel:* Diagram of the locations of bone resorption in the rat tibia during longitudinal growth (left). Effect of clodronate (right). *Lower panel:* Microradiograph of a normal tibia (left) and of a bone from an animal treated with clodronate (right). (Adapted from Schenk, R.K. *et al.* (1973). Reproduced from *Calcified Tissue Res.*, **11**, 196–214, with copyright permission from the author and Springer-Verlag, Heidelberg.)

The inhibition of bone resorption by bisphosphonates has also been documented using ^{45}Ca kinetic studies and hydroxyproline excretion, as well as by other means. The effect occurs within 24–48 h and is therefore slower than that of calcitonin.

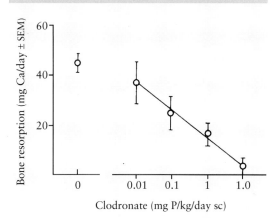

Fig. 2.3-5 Inhibition of bone resorption by subcutaneous (sc) administration of clodronate in the rat, as assessed by ^{45}Ca kinetics.

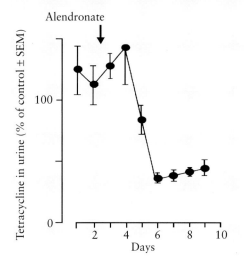

Fig. 2.3-6 Effect of one injection of 0.1 mg P/kg subcutaneously of alendronate on bone resorption, assessed by monitoring the urinary excretion of radioactive tetracycline from prelabeled rats. (Adapted from Mühlbauer, R.C. and Fleisch, H. (1990). A method for continuing monitoring of bone resorption in rats: evidence for a diurnal rhythm. *Am. J. Physiol.*, **259**, R679–R689, with permission from the authors and publisher.)

Bisphosphonates inhibit bone resorption in intact animals also.

The decrease in resorption is accompanied by an increase in calcium balance and in the mineral content of bone. This is possible because of an increase in intestinal calcium absorption, consequent on an elevation of 1,25(OH)$_2$ vitamin D. In growing rats treated over short periods, the

Calcium
balance
p. 23

increase in balance can reach 25%, but it is not known how long it ⟵
will be sustained. This increase is smaller than expected considering
the dramatic decrease in bone resorption. This is due to the fact that,
after a certain time, bone formation also decreases, because of the so-
called 'coupling' between formation and resorption. The main effect of
bisphosphonates is therefore a reduction in bone turnover. The increase
in balance is the basis for the administration of these compounds to prevent osteoporosis in humans.

Bisphos-
phonates in
osteoporosis
models
p. 128

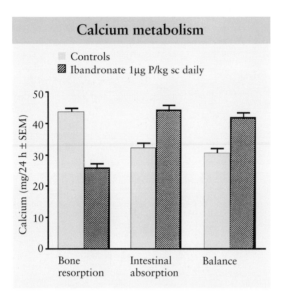

Fig. 2.3-7 Effect of
1 µg P/kg sc daily of ibandronate on calcium meta-
bolism in the rat. Bone
resorption was decreased
and calcium balance
increased.

Bisphosphonates increase calcium balance in normal animals.

Some studies have addressed the question of the effect of the bisphosphonates upon the mechanical properties of the skeleton. This issue is of
importance, since it is known that a long-lasting, strong inhibition of
bone resorption can lead to increased bone fragility both in animals and
in humans. This is well illustrated in the human osteopetrosis described
by Albers-Schönberg. Various studies have shown that bisphosphonates

Effect in
experimental
osteoporosis
p. 126

have a positive effect on mechanical characteristics, both in normal animals and in various experimental osteoporosis models. Bisphosphonates
proven to be active in this sense include alendronate, cimadronate, clodronate, etidronate, olpadronate, pamidronate, tiludronate and YH 529.

Chemistry of
bisphos-
phonates
pp. 35–36

However etidronate at high doses may induce an opposite effect, probably because of an inhibition of mineralization.

Animals with experimentally increased bone resorption

Bisphosphonates can also prevent experimentally induced increase in bone resorption. Thus, they impair resorption induced by agents such as parathyroid hormone, 1,25 (OH$_2$) vitamin D and retinoids, this effect having been used to develop a powerful and rapid screening assay for new compounds.

Fig. 2.3-8 Assessment of the action of inhibitors of bone resorption by means of retinoid-induced hypercalcemia in thyroparathyroidectomized rats.

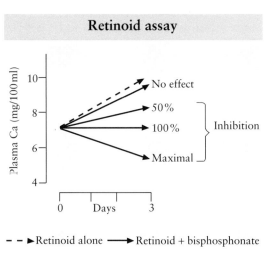

They also inhibit bone loss induced by different procedures such as immobilization, ovariectomy, corticosteroids and lactation under a low calcium diet. This aspect will be discussed in the section on osteoporosis in Chapter 3.

Osteoporosis models p. 125

Bisphosphonates also inhibit neoplastic bone resorption induced experimentally by implantation of various tumor cells. Both the actual destruction of bone by the invading tumor cells, and the resorption induced by systemically circulating factors, are slowed down. These effects lead to a total or partial prevention of hypercalcemia and hypercalciuria. This effect is the basis for their use in tumor bone disease.

Effect on experimental tumors p. 92

Of interest in the dental field is the fact that they also slow down periodontal bone destruction in rats susceptible to periodontal disease and in experimental periodontitis in monkeys.

Bisphosphonates very efficiently prevent experimentally induced bone resorption.

Relative activity of bisphosphonates

The activity of bisphosphonates on bone resorption varies greatly from compound to compound. For etidronate, the dose inhibiting resorption is relatively high, in the rat about 1 mg/kg parenterally per day. This dose is very near that which impairs normal mineralization. One of the aims of bisphosphonate research has therefore been to develop compounds with a more powerful antiresorptive activity, without a stronger inhibition of mineralization. This has proven to be possible. Clodronate was already more potent than etidronate, and pamidronate was found to be even more active. In recent years, compounds have been developed that are up to 10 000 times more powerful than etidronate in the inhibition of bone resorption in experimental animals without being more active in inhibiting mineralization.

Chemistry of bisphos-
phonates
pp. 35–36

Potency to inhibit bone resorption					
~1 ×	~10 ×	~100 ×	>100 – <1000 ×	>1000 – <10 000 ×	>10 000 ×
Etidronate	Clodronate Tiludronate	Pamidronate Neridronate	Alendronate Climadronate EB-1053 Olpadronate	Ibandronate Risedronate	YH 529 Zoledronate

Fig. 2.3-9 Potency of some bisphosphonates to inhibit bone resorption in the rat.

For the development of future compounds it is of relevance that, so far, the potency evaluated in the rat corresponds quite well with that found in humans.

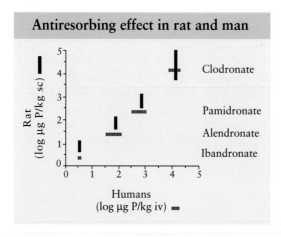

Fig. 2.3-10 Comparison of the dose of various bisphosphonates preventing retinoid-induced hypercalcemia in the rat, and the dose effective in tumoral hypercalcemia in humans. (Adapted from Mühlbauer, R.C. (1994). Reproduced from Ziegler, R., Pfeilschifter, J. and Bräutigam, M. (eds.) (1994). *Sex Steroids and Bone*, pp. 191–202, with permission from the author and Springer-Verlag, Heidelberg.)

*The potency of different bisphosphonates on bone resorption
varies from 1 for etidronate to approximately 10 000. There is a
good correlation between the potencies found in the rat and those
in humans.*

Up to now, no clear-cut structure–activity relationship has been
demonstrated. The length of the aliphatic carbon chain is important, the
effect on bone resorption increasing and then decreasing again with
increasing chain length. Adding a hydroxyl group to the carbon atom at
position 1 increases potency, and compounds with a nitrogen atom in the
side chains are extremely active. The first compound of this kind to be
described, pamidronate, has an amino group at the end of the side chain.
Again, the length of the side chain is relevant in these compounds, the
highest activity being found with a backbone of four carbons, as present
in alendronate. A primary amine is not necessary for this activity, as
dimethylation of the amino nitrogen of pamidronate, as seen in
olpadronate, increases efficacy. Activity can still be further increased
when other groups are added to the nitrogen, as is the case for example
in [1-hydroxy-3(methylpentylamino)propylidene]bis-phosphonate (ibandronate), which is extremely active.

Chemistry
of bisphos-
phonates
pp. 35–36

Cyclic geminal bisphosphonates are also very potent, especially those
containing a nitrogen atom in the ring, such as risedronate. The most
active compounds described so far, zoledronate and YH 529, belong to
this class and contain an imidazol ring.

It must be noted that at present, all effective compounds have a P-C-P
structure, which appears to be a prerequisite for activity. The intensity of
the effect is, however, dependent upon the side chain. Recent investigations showed that a three-dimensional structural requirement appears to
be involved. Indeed stereoisomers of the same chemical structure have
shown tenfold differences in activity. This opens the possibility of binding onto some kind of 'receptor'.

*No clear structure–effect relationship has yet emerged. The bind-
ing to the mineral appears to be due to the P-C-P structure,
while the antiresorptive activity is influenced by the structure of
the side chains and therefore the three-dimensional structure.*

A new approach to shorten the half-life in bone has been the synthesis
of new compounds, such as the phosphonoalkylphosphinates and the
phosphonocarboxylates, in which one of the phosphonate group is mod-
ified, so that it has a reduced affinity to the mineral.

Mechanisms of action

The mode of action of the bisphosphonates is still not completely eluci-dated. There is no doubt that the action *in vivo* is mediated mostly, if not completely, through mechanisms other than the physicochemical inhibi-tion of crystal dissolution, as was initially postulated. However, the nature of these mechanisms is still unclear and it may well be that more than one are operating at the same time.

There is a general consensus that the bisphosphonates act by inhibit-ing the activity of the osteoclasts. Indeed the morphology of osteoclasts is altered by bisphosphonates, both *in vitro* and *in vivo*.

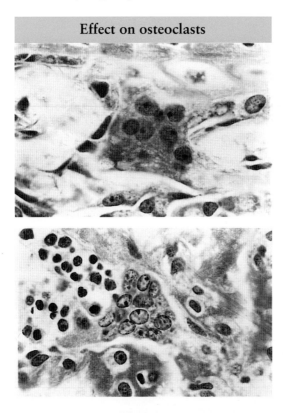

Effect on osteoclasts

Fig. 2.3-11 An osteoclast of a normal rat (above) and of an animal treated with a bisphosphonate (below). (Courtesy of Dr R.K. Schenk.)

Furthermore, the addition of bisphosphonates *in vitro* to osteoclasts exposed to mineralized substrata such as bone, dentine or ivory leads to inhibition of their resorbing activity. This activity is still present if these substrata are exposed to bisphosphonates before the osteoclasts are added. These results suggest that the osteoclasts are inhibited when they come into contact with bisphosphonate-containing bone. They support the hypothesis proposed for a long time, that bisphosphonates are deposited onto bone because of their strong affinity for the mineral, and that the osteoclasts are then inhibited when they start to engulf bisphosphonate-containing bone. This hypothesis is also supported by the recent finding that bisphosphonates, when administered in low amounts, deposit preferentially under the osteoclasts. It has been calculated that the bisphosphonate concentration below the osteoclasts can reach very high values. Lastly, this hypothesis would explain why a single administration of bisphosphonate can be active for a long period of time after discontinuation of the drug, both in animals and humans.

Duration of action in humans p. 97

Fig. 2.3-12 Mechanism of action of bisphosphonates: hypothesis 1. The osteoclast is inhibited directly after having taken up bisphosphonate from bone.

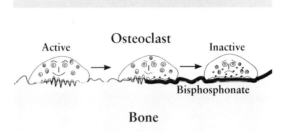

The biochemical mechanisms by which bisphosphonates inhibit osteoclasts are still unknown. A great number of different biochemical effects on various cell types have been described, but unfortunately only very few data exist on the osteoclasts themselves.

Fig. 2.3-13 Biochemical action of bisphosphonates on the osteoclast according to hypothesis 1.

Mode of action of bisphosphonates

Binding to apatite crystals
↓
Local release during bone resorption
Preferential accumulation under osteoclasts
↓
Decrease in osteoclast activity

- Acid production ↓
- Lysosomal and other enzymes ↓
- Prostaglandin formation ↓
- Membrame permeability ↑

Decrease in osteoclast number

- Recruitment ↓
- Apoptosis ↑

Some of these cellular effects may, however, be relevant to bone resorption, for example reduction in lactic acid production, proton secretion, reactive oxygen species production, lysosomal enzyme activity and prostaglandin synthesis, as well as changes in membrane permeability. Experiments on osteoclasts themselves have shown a change in membrane permeability, an inhibition of acid production, and an inhibition of the vacuolar-type proton ATPase present in the ruffled border. Very recently an inhibition of certain protein tyrosine phosphatases has been described. Lastly, the finding that an excellent correlation exists in a series of bisphosphonates, varying in activity by four orders of magnitude, between their inhibition of growth of the amoebae of a cellular slime mold and their inhibition of bone resorption *in vivo*, might lead to an interesting new path.

> *Bisphosphonates may directly affect the osteoclast when it dissolves bisphosphonate-coated mineral. The biochemical mechanisms of such an effect are still unknown, but appear to involve the acidification process at the ruffled border.*

Recent results, however, suggest that this mechanism might well not be the only one. Thus, it was found that bisphosphonates with up to a 1000-fold difference in activity in the living animal show, when added to the mineral, the same resorbing activity of osteoclasts *in vitro*. However, when the osteoclast population, which is invariably contaminated by other cells, especially osteoblasts, is exposed to the bisphosphonates before being added to the mineralized tissues, the activity is still present, but the potency of the various compounds now correlates well with that seen *in vivo*. These results suggest that resorption is inhibited even when the bisphosphonate is not taken up through the mineral, but is exposed directly to the cell suspension.

Effect of bisphosphonates *in vitro*

Bisphosphonate	50% inhibition *in vitro* (mol/l)	Relative potency *in vitro*	Relative potency *in vivo*
Etidronate	1×10^{-6}	1	1
Clodronate	1.5×10^{-7}	8	10
Pamidronate	3×10^{-9}	550	100
Alendronate	2×10^{-9}	700	700
Ibandronate	3.5×10^{-10}	5000	4000

Fig. 2.3-14 Effect of bisphosphonates *in vitro* after treatment of the osteoclast–osteoblast population before the latter was added to the mineral, compared to potency *in vivo* as assessed by the inhibition of retinoid-induced hypercalcemia. (Adapted from Sahni, M. *et al.* (1993). Reproduced from *J. Clin. Invest.*, 91, 2339–46, with copyright permission from the author and the American Society of Clinical Investigation.)

Bisphosphonates efficiently inhibit in vitro resorption of mineralized substrata even if they are added to cells only, but not to mineral. This casts doubt on the hypothesis that they must always act through binding onto mineral.

Later it was shown that the effect was not directly on the osteoclasts, but mediated through the osteoblasts, which are always present together with the osteoclasts. In the presence of concentrations of bisphosphonates as low as 10^{-10} to 10^{-11} mol/l, the osteoblasts secrete less osteoclast-stimulating activity, resulting in lower bone resorption. Very recently it has been shown that this decrease in activity is not due to a reduced production of an osteoblastic stimulator of resorption, but to the synthesis of an inhibitor of this process through an inhibition of osteoclast recruitment. An action through osteoblasts is possible since bisphosphonates can enter these cells, at least *in vitro*.

Fig. 2.3-15 Mechanism of action of bisphosphonates: hypothesis 2. The inhibition of the osteoclast is secondary to an increase in production by the osteoblast of an inhibitor of osteoclast recruitment or survival. The primary target is therefore the osteoblast.

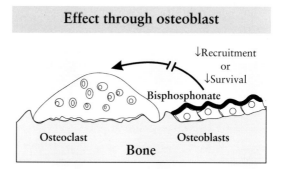

Bisphosphonates inhibit osteoclasts by stimulating the secretion of an inhibitor of osteoclast recruitment or survival by the osteoblasts. Therefore the target cell also appears to be the osteoblast.

It is not known at present which of the two mechanisms, the direct effect on the osteoclast or indirect action through the osteoblast, is operating *in vivo* and, if both are present, which of the two is more important.

It is not yet known which of the two mechanisms, the direct effect on the osteoclast or indirect action through the osteoblast, is more important in vivo.

The possibility that the decrease in resorption is also due to a decrease in the number of osteoclasts is supported by the fact that in humans chronic treatment often leads to a dramatic decrease in the number of osteoclasts. This can be either because cells already present are destroyed when they come into contact with bone containing the compounds, possibly because of apoptosis or because recruitment of new cells is inhibited. However, in the rat, the number of osteoclasts at the beginning of treatment is often increased, possibly secondary to an increase in histidine decarboxylase, in spite of the fact that bone resorption is blocked. Therefore, an effect through the recruitment or survival of osteoclasts may be present, but its importance is still unknown. It is possible that the first effect occurring in time is a direct one on the osteoclasts, while the more chronic action, when the number of osteoclasts is decreased, is mediated by the osteoblasts.

Bisphosphonates may also act by decreasing the number of osteoclasts, by inhibiting either their recruitment or their survival.

Lastly, macrophages are especially sensitive to bisphosphonates, which inhibit their activity and multiplication *in vitro*. This effect appears to be specific for the mononuclear phagocyte lineage. Since macrophages produce a variety of bone-resorbing cytokines, and as the osteoclasts originate from the monocyte phagocyte system, an effect through this pathway may also be postulated.

In view of the large array of their effects on cells, it is surprising that the bisphosphonates act almost exclusively on calcified tissues. This selectivity is explained by the strong affinity of these compounds for calcium phosphate, which allows them to be cleared very rapidly from blood and to be incorporated into calcified tissues, especially bone.

Pharmaco-
kinetics
p. 58

Bisphosphonates act specifically on bone, because of their affinity for bone mineral.

Inhibition of mineralization

Ectopic mineralization

Like pyrophosphate, bisphosphonates inhibit calcification *in vivo* very efficiently. Thus, they prevent experimentally induced calcification of many soft tissues such as arteries, kidneys, skin and heart. In contrast to pyrophosphate, which acts only when given parenterally, they are also active when administered orally. In the arteries they decrease not only mineral deposition, but also the accumulation of cholesterol, elastin and collagen.

Fig 2.3-16 Effect of 10 mg P/kg body weight of bisphosphonates on vitamin D_3-induced aortic calcification in the rat. Subcutaneous (sc) compared with oral (po) administration. (Adapted from Fleisch, H. *et al.* (1970). Reproduced with permission from the author and the publisher.)

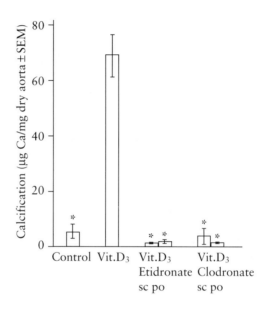

A possibly interesting future use of bisphosphonates could arise from the finding that some of them, such as etidronate, can also inhibit the calcification of bioprosthetic heart valves, either when administered subcutaneously or when released locally from various matrices. Investigations are in progress to bind bisphosphonates covalently to the valves.

Certain bisphosphonates like etidronate also decrease the formation of experimental urinary stones and inhibit ectopic calcification and ossification, the latter when given either systemically or locally. This effect has led to the clinical use of etidronate in ectopic ossification. However, normal mineralization is inhibited as well. Lastly, topical administration of etidronate leads to a decreased formation of dental calculus.

Use in ectopic calcification and ossification pp. 140–143

Bisphosphonates in vivo inhibit experimentally induced soft tissue calcification and ossification, urinary stones and dental calculus.

Normal mineralization

The dose, at least of etidronate, which inhibits experimental ectopic min- ←
eralization, also impairs the mineralization of normal calcified tissues
such as bone, cartilage, dentine and enamel. The amount required to
have this effect varies according to the animal species and the length of
treatment. In contrast to bone resorption, where the different compounds vary greatly in their activity, this does not seem to be so much the
case for the inhibition of mineralization. For most species, the effective
daily dose is in the order of 5–20 mg of compound phosphorus per kg.
Interestingly, clodronate inhibits normal mineralization somewhat less
than does etidronate, despite the fact that it is more active on bone
resorption. This may be due to the fact that clodronate has no hydroxyl
side chain and is therefore less bound to the mineral. The inhibition of
calcification with high doses can lead to fractures and to an impairment

Adverse
events
pp. 148–150

of fracture healing. The effect on mineralization is eventually reversed
after discontinuation of the drug. Nevertheless, the propensity to inhibit
the mineralization of ectopic calcification of normal bone has hampered

Heterotopic
calcification
and
ossification
p. 140–143

the therapeutic use of bisphosphonates in ectopic calcification. This is
not the case for their use in bone resorption, since compounds have been
developed that inhibit this process at 1000 times lower doses than the
one that inhibits mineralization.

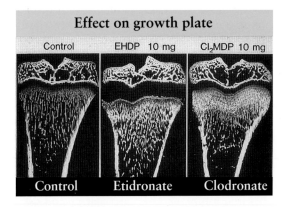

Fig. 2.3-17 Inhibition of ←
mineralization of bone and
cartilage in the growing
rat by 10 mg P/kg subcutaneously of etidronate but
not clodronate daily
for 7 days. (Courtesy of
Dr R.K. Schenk.)

*Bisphosphonates, if given at high doses, inhibit the mineralization
of normal calcified tissues inducing rickets and osteomalacia.
While this is a problem in humans when it is used to prevent
ectopic calcification or ossification, it is not the case for most
bisphosphonates when they are used to decrease bone resorption.*

Mechanisms of action

There is a close relationship between the ability of an individual bisphosphonate to inhibit the formation of calcium phosphate *in vitro* and its effectiveness on calcification *in vivo*, strongly suggesting that the latter can be explained in terms of a physicochemical mechanism. However, an additional effect on matrix formation cannot be excluded, since changes in glycosaminoglycan and collagen synthesis have been found.

Physico-chemical effects p. 38

> *The inhibition of mineralization* in vivo, *both on normal and ectopic calcification, is probably explained by a physicochemical mechanism.*

Other effects

Another interesting finding is that bisphosphonates, among others risedronate, inhibit local bone resorption, preserve the joint architecture and decrease the inflammatory reaction in experimental arthritis induced by Freund's adjuvant. Furthermore, clodronate and other new bisphosphonates also inhibit the delayed-type hypersensitivity granuloma response. Moreover, bisphosphonates or phosphonosulfonates linked to an isoprene chain are potent inhibitors of squalene synthase and hence cholesterol-lowering agents in the animal. These results may open some interesting new therapeutic possibilities for these drugs.

→ Lastly, it is worth mentioning that bisphosphonates were found at very low concentrations to increase colony formation, mineralization and osteocalcin synthesis in bone cell cultures *in vitro*. This result would strengthen the suggestion often made, but never proven, that bisphosphonates might, in certain conditions, increase bone formation *in vivo*. However, this theory still needs to be verified.

Recommended selected reading

Reviews

Bauss, F. and Mühlbauer, R.C. (1994). BM 21.0955, monosodium salt, monohydrate. *Drugs Fut.*, **19**, 13–16

Fleisch, H. (1988). Bisphosphonates: a new class of drugs in diseases of bone and calcium metabolism. In Baker, P.F. (ed.) *Handbook of Experimental Pharmacology*, vol. 83, pp. 441–66. (Berlin, Heidelberg: Springer-Verlag)

Fleisch, H. (1993). Bisphosphonates: mechanisms of action and clinical use. In Mundy, G.R. and Martin, T.J. (eds.) *Physiology and Pharmacology of Bone. Handbook of Experimental Pharmacology*, vol. 107, pp. 377–418. (Berlin, Heidelberg, New York: Springer-Verlag)

Geddes, A.D., D'Souza, S.M., Ebetino, F.H. and Ibbotson, K.J. (1994). Bisphosphonates: structure–activity relationships and therapeutic implications. In Heersche, J.N.M. and Kanis, J.A. (eds.) *Bone and Mineral Research*, pp. 265–306. (Amsterdam, London, New York, Tokyo: Elsevier)

Reginster, J.Y.L. (1992). Oral tiludronate: pharmacological properties and potential usefulness in Paget's disease of bone and osteoporosis. *Bone*, 13, 351–4

Original articles

Physical chemistry

Fleisch, H., Russell, R.G.G., Bisaz, S., Mühlbauer, R.C. and Williams, D.A. (1970). The inhibitory effect of phosphonates on the formation of calcium phosphate crystals *in vitro* and on aortic and kidney calcification *in vivo*. *Eur. J. Clin. Invest.*, 1, 12–18

Francis, M.D. (1969). The inhibition of calcium hydroxyapatite crystal growth by polyphosphonates and polyphosphates. *Calcif. Tissue Res.*, 3, 151–62

Jung, A., Bisaz, S. and Fleisch, H. (1973). The binding of pyrophosphate and two diphosphonates by hydroxyapatite crystals. *Calcif. Tissue Res.*, 11, 269–80

Russell, R.G.G., Mühlbauer, R.C., Bisaz, S., Williams, D.A. and Fleisch, H. (1970). The influence of pyrophosphate, condensed phosphates, phosphonates and other phosphate compounds on the dissolution of hydroxyapatite *in vitro* and on bone resorption induced by parathyroid hormone in tissue culture and in thyroparathyroidectomised rats. *Calcif. Tissue Res.*, 6, 183–96

Mineralization

Briner, W.W., Francis, M.D. and Widder, J.S. (1971). The control of dental calculus in experimental animals. *Int. Dent. J.*, 21, 61–73

Fleisch, H., Russell, R.G.G., Bisaz, S., Mühlbauer, R.C. and Williams, D.A. (1970). The inhibitory effect of phosphonates on the formation of calcium phosphate crystals *in vitro* and on aortic and kidney calcification *in vivo*. *Eur. J. Clin. Invest.*, 1, 12–18

Francis, M.D., Russell, R.G.G. and Fleisch, H. (1969). Diphosphonates inhibit formation of calcium phosphate crystals *in vitro* and pathological calcification *in vivo*. *Science*, 165, 1264–6

King, W.R., Francis, M.D. and Michael, W.R. (1971). Effect of disodium ethane-1-hydroxy-1,1-diphosphonate on bone formation. *Clin. Orthop.*, 78, 251–70

Schenk, R., Merz, W.A., Mühlbauer, R., Russell, R.G.G. and Fleisch, H. (1973). Effect of ethane-1-hydroxy-1,1-diphosphonate (EHDP) and dichloromethylene diphosphonate (Cl_2MDP) on the calcification and resorption of cartilage and bone in the tibial epiphysis and metaphysis of rats. *Calcif. Tissue Res.*, 11, 196–214

Shinoda, H., Adamek, G., Felix, R., Fleisch, H., Schenk, R. and Hagan, P. (1983). Structure–activity relationships of various bisphosphonates. *Calcif. Tissue Int.*, 35, 87–99

Bone resorption

Ferretti, J.L., Cointry, G., Capozza, R., Montuori, E., Roldán, E. and Pérez Lloret, A. (1990). Biomechanical effects of the full range of useful doses of (3-amino-1-hydroxypropylidene)-1,1-bisphosphonate (APD) on femur diaphyses and cortical bone tissue in rats. *Bone Miner.*, 11: 111–22

Fleisch, H., Russell, R.G.G. and Francis, M.D. (1969). Diphosphonates inhibit hydroxy-apatite dissolution *in vitro* and bone resorption in tissue culture and *in vivo*. *Science*, **165**, 1262–4

Gasser, A.B., Morgan, D.B., Fleisch, H.A. and Richelle, L.J. (1972). The influence of two diphosphonates on calcium metabolism in the rat. *Clin. Sci.*, **43**, 31–45

Geusens, P., Nijs, J., van der Perre, G., van Audekercke, R., Lowet, G., Goovaerts, S., Barbier, A., Lacheretz, F., Remandet, B., Jiang, Y. and Dequeker, J. (1992). Longitudinal effect of tiludronate on bone mineral density, resonant frequency, and strength in monkeys. *J. Bone Miner. Res.*, **7**, 599–609

Green, J.R., Müller, K. and Jaeggi, K.A. (1994). Preclinical pharmacology of CGP 42'446, a new, potent, heterocyclic bisphosphonate compound. *J. Bone Miner. Res.*, **9**, 745–51

Guy, J.A., Shea, M., Peter, C.P., Morrissey, R. and Hayes, W.C. (1993). Continuous alen-dronate treatment throughout growth, maturation, and aging in the rat results in increases in bone mass and mechanical properties. *Calcif. Tissue Int.*, **53**, 283–8

Mühlbauer, R.C., Bauss, F., Schenk, R., Janner, M., Bosies, E., Strein, K. and Fleisch, H. (1991). BM 21.0955, a potent new bisphosphonate to inhibit bone resorption. *J. Bone Miner. Res.*, **6**: 1003–11

Reitsma, P.H., Bijvoet, O.L.M., Verlinden-Ooms, H. and van der Wee-Pals, L.J.A. (1980). Kinetic studies of bone and mineral metabolism during treatment with (3-amino-1-hydroxypropylidene)-1,1-bisphosphonate (ADP) in rats. *Calcif. Tissue Int.*, **32**, 145–57

Reynolds, J.J., Minkin, C., Morgan, D.B., Spycher, D. and Fleisch, H. (1972). The effect of two diphosphonates on the resorption of mouse calvaria *in vitro*. *Calcif. Tissue Res.*, **10**, 302–13

Reynolds, J.J., Murphy, H., Mühlbauer, R.C., Morgan, D.B. and Fleisch, H. (1973). Inhibition by diphosphonates of bone resorption in mice and comparison with grey-lethal osteopetrosis. *Calcif. Tissue Res.*, **12**, 59–71

Rogers, M.J., Watts, D.J., Russell, R.G.G., Ji, X., Xiong, X., Blackburn, G.M., Bayless, A.V. and Ebetino, F.H. (1994). Inhibitory effects of bisphosphonates on growth of amoebae of the cellular slime mold dictostelium discoideum. *J. Bone Miner. Res.*, **9**, 1029–39

Russell, R.G.G., Mühlbauer, R.C., Bisaz, S., Williams, D.A. and Fleisch, H. (1970). The influence of pyrophosphate, condensed phosphates, phosphonates and other phosphate compounds on the dissolution of hydroxyapatite *in vitro* and on bone resorption induced by parathyroid hormone in tissue culture and in thyroparathyroidectomised rats. *Calcif. Tissue Res.*, **6**, 183–96

Schenk, R., Eggli, P., Fleisch, H. and Rosini, S. (1986). Quantitative morphometric evalua-tion of the inhibitory activity of new aminobisphosphonates on bone resorption in the rat. *Calcif. Tissue Int.*, **38**, 342–9

Trechsel, U., Stutzer, A. and Fleisch, H. (1987). Hypercalcemia induced with an arotinoid in thyroparathyroidectomized rats. New model to study bone resorption in vivo. *J. Clin. Invest.*, **80**, 1679–86

van der Pluijm, G., Binderup, L., Bramm, E., van der Wee-Pals, L., de Groot, H., Binderup, E., Löwik, C. and Papapoulos, S. (1992). Disodium 1-hydroxy-3-(1-pyrrolidinyl)-propylidene-1,1-bisphosphonate (EB-1053) is a potent inhibitor of bone resorption *in vitro* and *in vivo*. *J. Bone Miner. Res.*, **7**, 981–6

Other effects

Ciosek, C. P., Magnin, D. R., Harrity, T. W. *et al.* (1993). Lipophilic 1, 1-bisphosphonates are potent squalene synthase inhibitors and orally active cholesterol lowering agents *in vivo*. *J. Biol. Chem.*, **268**, 24832–7

Dunn, C.J., Galinet, L.A., Wu, H., Nugent, R.A., Schlachter, S.T., Staite, N.D., Aspar, D.G., Elliott, G.A., Essani, N.A., Rohloff, N.A. and Smith, R.J. (1993). Demonstration of novel anti-arthritic and anti-inflammatory effects of diphosphonates. *J. Pharmacol. Exp. Ther.*, **266**, 1691–8

Endo, Y., Nakamura, M., Kikuchi, T., Shinoda, H., Takeda, Y., Nitta, Y, and Kumagai, K. (1993). Aminoalkylbisphosphonates, potent inhibitors of bone resorption, induce a prolonged stimulation of histamine synthesis and increase machrophages, granulocytes, and osteoclasts *in vivo*. *Calcif. Tissue Int.*, **52**, 248–54

Francis, M.D., Hovancik, K. and Boyce, R.W. (1989). NE-58095: a diphosphonate which prevents bone erosion and preserves joint architecture in experimental arthritis. *Int. J. Tissue React.*, **11**, 239–52

Österman, T., Kippo, K., Laurén, L., Hannuniemi, R. and Sellman, R. (1994). Effect of clodronate on established adjuvant arthritis. *Rheumatol. Int.*, **14**, 139–47

Tsuchimoto, M., Azuma, Y., Higuchi, O., Sugimoto, I., Hirata, N., Kiyoki, M. and Yamamoto, I. (1994). Alendronate modulates osteogenesis of human osteoblastic cells *in vitro*. *Jpn. J. Pharmacol.*, **66**, 25–33

Mechanisms

Boonekamp, P.M., van der Wee-Pals, L.J.A., van Wijk-van Lennep, M.M.L., Thesing, C.W. and Bijvoet, O.L.M. (1986). Two modes of action of bisphosphonates on osteoclastic resorption of mineralized matrix. *Bone Miner.*, **1**, 27–39

Carano, A., Teitelbaum, S.L., Konsek, J.D., Schlesinger, P.H. and Blair, H.C. (1990). Bisphosphonates directly inhibit the bone resorption activity of isolated avian osteoclasts *in vitro*. *J. Clin. Invest.*, **85**, 456–61

Fast, D.K., Felix, R., Dowse, C., Neuman, W.F. and Fleisch, H. (1978). The effects of diphosphonates on the growth and glycolysis of connective-tissue cells in culture. *Biochem. J.*, **172**, 97–107

Felix, R., Bettex, J.D. and Fleisch, H. (1981). Effect of diphosphonates on the synthesis of prostaglandins in cultured calvaria cells. *Calcif. Tissue Int.*, **33**, 549–52

Felix, R., Russell, R.G.G. and Fleisch, H. (1976). The effect of several diphosphonates on acid phosphohydrolases and other lysosomal enzymes. *Biochim. Biophys. Acta*, **429**, 429–38

Flanagan, A.M. and Chambers, T.J. (1989). Dichloromethylenebisphosphonate (Cl$_2$MBP) inhibits bone resorption through injury to osteoclasts that resorb Cl$_2$MBP-coated bone. *Bone Miner.*, **6**, 33–43

Sahni, M., Guenther, H.L., Fleisch, H., Collin, P. and Martin, T.J. (1993). Bisphosphonates act on rat bone resorption through the mediation of osteoblasts. *J. Clin. Invest.*, **91**, 2004–11

Sato, M. and Grasser, W. (1990). Effects of bisphosphonates on isolated rat osteoclasts as examined by reflected light microscopy. *J. Bone Miner. Res.*, **5**, 31–40

Sato, M., Grasser, W., Endo, N., Akins, R., Simmons, H., Thompson, D.D., Golub, E. and Rodan, G.A. (1991). Bisphosponate action. Alendronate localization in rat bone and effects on osteoclast ultrastructure. *J. Clin. Invest.*, **88**, 2095–105

2.4. PHARMACOKINETICS

Bisphosphonates are synthetic compounds, which have not yet been found to occur naturally in animals or humans. No enzymes able to cleave the P-C-P bonds have been described. The bisphosphonates on which data have been published so far, i.e. alendronate, clodronate, etidronate, pamidronate and tiludronate, appear to be absorbed, stored and excreted unaltered from the body. Therefore, these bisphosphonates seem to be non-biodegradable, in solution and in animals. However, it cannot be excluded that other bisphosphonates may be metabolized, especially in their side chains.

Bisphosphonates are not biodegradable.

Data from relatively few pharmacokinetic studies are available. Most of the data have been obtained with alendronate, clodronate, etidronate, pamidronate and tiludronate.

2.4.1. Intestinal absorption

→ The bioavailability of an oral dose of a bisphosphonate in animals as well as in humans is low, between less than 1% and 10%. It is generally lower for the more potent bisphosphonates, such as the amino derivatives, which are administered in lower amounts. It is in general higher in the young and shows great inter- and intraspecies variation. This variability represents a problem in humans, especially for compounds like etidronate, where the dose that inhibits resorption is close to that which inhibits mineralization. Absorption occurs to some extent in the stomach and to a larger extent in the small intestine. It appears to occur by passive diffusion, possibly through a paracellular pathway. It is diminished when the drug is given with meals, especially in the presence of calcium and iron. The mechanism of this inhibition may be due to the conversion of the bisphosphonate into a non-absorbable form, or to a decrease of the absorption process itself. Therefore, bisphosphonates should never be given at mealtimes and never together with milk or dairy products or with iron supplements. Also, orange juice and coffee decrease absorbtion.

Inhibition of mineralization pp. 148–150

Bisphosphonates are poorly absorbed, especially in the presence of calcium.

2.4.2. Distribution

In the blood, about two-thirds or more of etidronate and clodronate, half ← of pamidronate, but much less of some others such as alendronate, are ultrafilterable. These values are strongly species-dependent. The remainder is either bound to proteins, especially albumin, or present in very small aggregates. Up to 60% or more of the absorbed bisphosphonate is then taken up by bone, the remainder being rapidly excreted in the urine. The uptake varies with species, sex and age and with the compound. In humans the values are about 20% for clodronate, 50% for etidronate and more for alendronate and pamidronate. Sometimes bisphosphonates, especially pamidronate, can deposit in other organs, mostly the liver and the spleen. The deposition is proportionally greater when large amounts of the compounds are given. Part of this extraosseous deposition appears to be due to the formation of complexes with metals or to aggregates after too high or too rapid intravenous injection. These complexes are then phagocytosed by the macrophages of the reticulo-endothelial system. Therefore, data obtained from studies using large amounts of labeled bisphosphonate given rapidly intravenously should be interpreted with caution. The formation of aggregates in the blood is thought to occur in humans following rapid intravenous injections of large quantities, possibly explaining the renal failure that can ensue.

Adverse events
p. 146

> *Bisphosphonates should not be infused rapidly in large quantities, as this can cause the formation of insoluble aggregates or complexes.*

The half-life of circulating bisphosphonates is short, in the rat of the order of minutes. In humans it is somewhat longer, 0.5–2 h. The rate of entry into bone is very fast, similar to that of calcium and phosphate. ← Bone clearance can be compatible with a complete extraction by the skeleton after the first passage, so that skeletal uptake might be determined to a large extent by its vascularization. The areas of deposition are generally thought to be mostly those of bone formation. This property is used to measure areas of high bone turnover in nuclear medicine by means of ^{99m}Tc-linked bisphosphonates. Recently, however, alendronate, when given in therapeutic doses, has been found to accumulate preferentially under the osteoclasts. This is also the case, although to a lesser extent, for etidronate when given in the same amount. When given at a therapeutic dose, the latter, however, accumulates equally under both cells. The rapid uptake by bone means that the soft tissues are exposed to bisphosphonates for only short periods, explaining why practically only bone is affected *in vivo*.

Bisphosphonates deposit rapidly into bone, in areas of both bone formation and bone destruction. The half-life in plasma is therefore very short.

When bisphosphonates are given in clinically effective doses, there seems to be no saturation in their total skeletal uptake in humans, at least within periods as long as years or decades. In contrast, with continuous administration, the antiresorbing effect reaches a maximum relatively rapidly, both in animals and in man. The level of this maximal effect depends upon the dose administered, as does the duration of the effect after discontinuation of the drug. The cause of this discrepancy between the time required for the maximal incorporation of the drug and that required for its maximal effect is not clear, but may reside in the unequal distribution within the skeleton. The fact that a plateau of activity is reached, despite the fact that the bisphosphonate continues to be incorporated, suggests also that the compound is buried in the bone and becomes inactive.

Effect in man
p. 132

Fig. 2.4-1 Effect of various doses of pamidronate on urinary hydroxyproline excretion in the rat. The maximal effect is obtained rapidly and depends upon the dose given. (Adapted and reproduced from Reitsma, P.H. *et al.* (1980). *Cacif. Tissue Int.*, **32**, 145–57, with copyright permission from the author and Springer-Verlag, Heidelberg.)

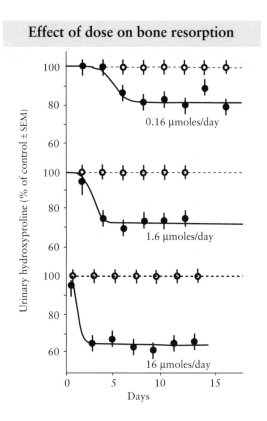

Effect of dose on bone resorption

Urinary hydroxyproline (% of control ± SEM)

0.16 µmoles/day

1.6 µmoles/day

16 µmoles/day

Days

The accumulation in the skeleton reaches a plateau with chronic administration only after a very long time, possibly decades. In contrast, the plateau of the effect is attained more rapidly and is dose-dependent.

Once buried in the skeleton under new layers of bone, the bisphosphonates are liberated again, some by physicochemical mechanisms, but mostly when the bone in which they were deposited is resorbed. Thus the half-life in the body depends to a large extent upon the rate of bone turnover itself. As the bisphosphonates slow down the resorption of the bone in which they are deposited, their half-life may be even longer than the normal half-life of the skeleton. The half-life of various bisphosphonates is between 3 months and up to a year in mice or rats, clodronate being cleared somewhat faster than etidronate and pamidronate. For humans it is much longer, and it is possible that part of the administered bisphosphonates remains in the body for life. However, this is also true for other 'bone seekers' such as tetracyclines and fluoride.

There is no indication that the bisphosphonate buried in the skeleton has any pharmacological activity. On the contrary, recent data indicate that in the rat, bone formed under administration of even high doses of alendronate can be resorbed normally. If, however, it is still active, the long skeletal retention may explain why one single administration of a bisphosphonate can be active for long periods of time, both in animals and in humans.

Tumor hyper-
calcemia
p. 97
Paget's disease
p. 75

The skeletal retention of bisphosphonates is very long, possibly life-long.

2.4.3. Renal clearance

The renal clearance of bisphosphonates is high. When taking into ← account their only partial ultrafilterability, it can be around that of inulin or even higher, as shown for alendronate. This high clearance suggests the presence of a renal secretory pathway (*see* Fig. 2.4-2).

2.4.4. Other modes of application

Recently it has been found that bisphosphonates are also bioavailable when given intranasally and through the skin. This opens new modes of administration in clinical practice.

Fig. 2.4-2 Pharmacokinetics of bisphosphonates.

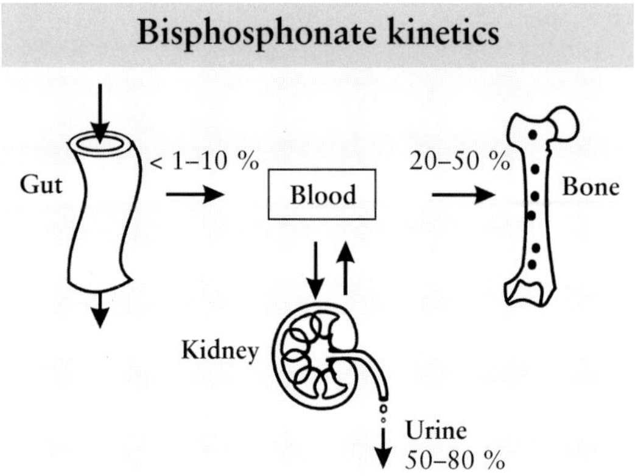

Recommended selected reading

Review

Fleisch, H. (1991). Bisphosphonates. Pharmacology and use in the treatment of tumour-induced hypercalcaemic and metastatic bone disease. *Drugs*, **42**, 919–44

Original articles

Bisaz, S., Jung, A. and Fleisch, H. (1978). Uptake by bone of pyrophosphate, diphosphonates and their technetium derivatives. *Clin. Sci. Mol. Med.*, **54**, 265–72

Boulenc, X., Marti, E., Joyeux, H., Roques, C., Berger, Y. and Fabre, G. (1993). Importance of the paracellular pathway for the transport of new bisphophonate using the human CACO-2 monolayers model. *Biochem. Pharmacol.*, **46** (9), 1591–600

Cheung, W.K., Brunner, L., Schoenfeld, S., Knight, R., Seaman, J., Brox, A., Batist, G., John, V. and Chan, K. (1994). Pharmacokinetics of pamidronate disodium in cancer patients after a single intravenous infusion of 30- , 60- or 90-mg dose over 4 or 24 hours. *Am. J. Therap.*, **1**, 288–35

Conrad, K.A. and Lee, S.M. (1981). Clodronate kinetics and dynamics. *Clin. Pharmacol. Ther.*, **30**, 114–20

Daley-Yates, P.T., Dodwell, D.J., Pongchaidecha, M., Coleman, R.E. and Howell, A. (1991). The clearance and bioavailability of pamidronate in patients with breast cancer and bone metastases. *Calcif. Tissue Int.*, **49**, 433–5

Gertz, B.J., Holland, S.D., Kline, W.F., Matuszewski, B.K. and Porras, A.G. (1993). Clinical pharmacology of alendronate sodium. *Osteoporosis Int.* (Suppl. 3), S13–16

Gural, R.P. (1975). *Pharmacokinetics and Gastrointestinal Absorption Behavior of Etridronate*. Dissertation, University of Kentucky

Gural, R.P., Chungi, V.S., Shrewsbury, R.P. and Dittert L.W. (1985). Dose-dependent absorption of disodium etidronate. *J. Pharm. Pharmacol.*, **37**, 443–5

Hanhijärvi, H., Elomaa, I., Karlsson, M. and Lauren, L. (1989). Pharmacokinetics of disodium clodronate after daily intravenous infusions during five consecutive days. *Int. J. Clin. Pharmacol. Ther. Toxicol.*, **27**, 602–6

Hyldstrup, L., Flesch, G. and Hauffe, S.A. (1993). Pharmacokinetic evaluation of pamidronate after oral administration: a study on dose proportionality, absolute bioavailability, and effect of repeated administration. *Calcif. Tissue Int.*, **53**, 297–300

Kasting, G.B. and Francis, M.D. (1992). Retention of etidronate in human, dog and rat. *J. Bone Miner. Res.*, **7**, 513–22

Lin, J.H., Chen, I.-W. and Duggan, D.E. (1992). Effects of dose, sex, and age on the disposition of alendronate, a potent antiosteolytic bisphosphonate, in rats. *Drug Metab. Dispos.*, **20**, 473–8

Lin, J.H., Chen, I.-W., Florencia, A., Deluna, A. and Hichens, M. (1992). Renal handling of alendronate in rats: an uncharacterized renal transport system. *Drug Metab. Dispos.*, **20**, 608–13

Michael, W.R., King, W.R. and Wakim, J.M. (1972). Metabolism of disodium ethane-1-hydroxy-1,1-diphosphonate (disodium etidronate) in the rat, rabbit, dog and monkey. *Toxicol. Appl. Pharmacol.*, **21**, 503–15

Mönkkönen, J., Koponen, H.M. and Ylitalo, P. (1990). Comparison of the distribution of three bisphosphonates in mice. *Pharmacol. Toxicol.*, **66**, 294–8

O'Rourke, N.P., McCloskey, E.V., Neugebauer, G. and Kanis, J.A. (1994). Renal and non-renal clearance of clodronate in patients with malignancy and renal impairment. *Drug Invest.*, **7**, 26–33

Österman, T., Juhakoski, A., Laurén, L. and Sellman, R. (1994). Effect of iron on the absorption and distribution of clodronate after oral administration in rats. *Pharmacol Toxicol.*, **74**, 267–70

Pongchaidecha, M. and Daley-Yates, P.T. (1993). Clearance and tissue uptake following 4-hour and 24-hour infusions of pamidronate in rats. *Drug Metab. Dispos.*, **21**, 100–3

Powell, J.H. and DeMark, B.R. (1985). Clinical pharmacokinetics of diphosphonates. In Garattini, S. (ed.) *Bone Resorption, Metastasis, and Diphosphonates*, pp. 41–9. (New York: Raven Press)

Recker, R.R. and Saville, P.D. (1973). Intestinal absorption of disodium ethane-1-hydroxy-1,1-diphosphonate (disodium etidronate) using a deconvolution technique. *Toxicol. Appl. Pharmacol.*, **24**, 580–9

Troehler, U., Bonjour, J.P. and Fleisch, H. (1975). Renal secretion of diphosphonates in rats. *Kidney Int.*, **8**, 6–13

Wingen, F. and Schmähl, D. (1987). Pharmacokinetics of the osteotropic diphosphonate 3-amino-1-hydroxypropane-1, 1-diphosphonic acid in mammals. *Arzneimittelforschung*, **37**, 1037–42

Yakatan, G.J., Poynor, W.J., Talbert, R.L., Floyd, B.F., Slough, C.L., Ampulski, R.S. and Benedict, J.J. (1982). Clodronate kinetics and bioavailability. *Clin. Pharmacol. Ther.*, **31**, 402–10

2.5. Animal toxicology

Published animal toxicological data are scanty and deal almost exclusively with alendronate, clodronate, etidronate, pamidronate and tiludronate. Unfortunately, practically nothing is published about other compounds.

Acute, subacute and chronic administration in several animal species have in general revealed little toxicity. Teratogenicity, mitogenicity and carcinogenicity tests have been negative. When these compounds are administered subcutaneously, local toxicity can occur, with local necrosis. This is especially the case for the amino derivatives such as pamidronate.

2.5.1. Acute toxicity

Acute toxicity presents the clinical picture of hypocalcemia and appears to be due mainly to the formation of complexes or aggregates with calcium, which lead to a decrease in ionized calcium. Toxicity therefore varies with the speed of infusion when the compounds are administered intravenously, so that the rate of infusion in humans must be carefully controlled. In the event of hypocalcemia, calcium infusion can rapidly correct the signs and symptoms.

Infusion in humans p. 146

Acute toxicity is due to hypocalcemia.

2.5.2. Non-acute toxicity

In view of the large array of cellular effects obtained *in vitro* with the bisphosphonates, one would have expected a large number of toxic effects. This is not the case, and when administered in pharmacological doses, the bisphosphonates seem to act almost exclusively on calcified tissues, and secondarily on calcemia. This selectivity is explained by the strong affinity of these compounds for calcium phosphate, which allows them to be rapidly incorporated into these tissues, especially bone, and therefore to be cleared quickly from the blood.

Pharmaco-kinetics p. 58

Bisphosphonates have low toxicity. They act specifically on bone, because of their affinity for bone mineral.

The non-skeletal toxicity associated with the compounds used clinically occurs only when doses substantially larger than those which inhibit bone resorption are used. In general, the first organ to show cellular alterations with all bisphosphonates, as well as with polyphosphates and phosphate itself, is the kidney. The liver can in some cases also show alterations. Some inflammatory gastrointestinal changes have been described. Developmental disturbances of enamel can also appear at high systemic doses. Lastly, at least certain bisphosphonates, such as etidronate and pamidronate, cross the placenta and can affect the fetus.

> *The first organ, apart from bone, to show alterations is the kidney. At least some bisphosphonates can cross the placenta and affect the fetus.*

It must be stressed that the results with one bisphosphonate cannot necessarily be extrapolated to other bisphosphonates. Indeed toxicity, both in cell and organ culture and *in vivo*, varies greatly from one compound to another.

> *Toxicity varies greatly from one bisphosphonate to another.*

Clodronate

Clodronate is well tolerated. Inhibition of mineralization can occur, but requires higher doses than with etidronate. At high doses, fractures can occur, without signs of osteomalacia or rickets. The fractures are probably caused by the long-term decrease in bone turnover, which can itself lead to an increased fragility, as is well known in human congenital osteopetrosis.

Kidney alterations are seen at high doses, and with very high doses atrophy of the thymus and some immunological alterations can occur in newborn animals.

Six-month toxicology studies with clodronate have shown that a daily oral amount of 200 mg/kg and 40 mg/kg are the highest non-toxic doses in the rat and dog, respectively.

> *Clodronate is in general well tolerated.*

Etidronate

Etidronate is generally well tolerated. The most relevant toxicity associated with this bisphosphonate is the inhibition of bone calcification. This starts to occur at doses of approximately 10 mg/kg daily. The picture looks radiologically like rickets or osteomalacia, although there are some histological differences. Fractures can occur after long-term administration which may be due to both the defective mineralization and the decrease in turnover. Renal lesions can be induced with high doses.

Inhibition of mineralization p. 52

Very large doses (200 mg/kg subcutaneously) of etidronate, given to pregnant rats, that is about 300 times the maximal oral dose of 20 mg/kg used in humans, lead to fetal abnormalities of the skeleton and the skin and induce malformations and hemorrhages.

Etidronate is in general well tolerated. The most relevant toxicity associated with etidronate is an inhibition of the mineralization of calcified tissues. At higher doses renal lesions appear, as is generally the case for bisphosphonates.

Pamidronate

Pamidronate also can lead to kidney alterations, the safety margin between the toxic dose and that inhibiting bone resorption being somewhat smaller than with etidronate and clodronate. Large doses of pamidronate (60 mg/kg per day and more orally) can decrease the number of live pups and pup viability in rats. Intravenous administration of 1 mg/kg per day and more produce alterations in the skeleton and kidney of the offspring.

Other bisphosphonates

A toxic dose of cimadronate has induced in the dog the formation of immature woven bone in the marrow of various bones. This observation, which has not yet had an explanation is an unique finding in the field of bisphosphonates.

Recommended selected reading

Reviews

Fleisch, H. (1991). Bisphosphonates. Pharmacology and use in the treatment of tumour-induced hypercalcaemic and metastatic bone disease. *Drugs*, **42**, 919–44
Reginster, J.Y.L. (1992). Oral tiludronate: pharmacological properties and potential usefulness in Paget's disease of bone and osteoporosis. *Bone*, **13**, 351–4

Original articles

Alden, C.L., Parker, R.D. and Eastman, D.F. (1989). Development of an acute model for the study of chloromethanediphosphonate nephrotoxicity. *Toxicol. Pathol.*, **17**, 27–32
Cal, J.C. and Daley-Yates, P.T. (1990). Disposition and nephrotoxicity of 3-amino-1-hydroxypropylidene-1,1-bisphosphonate (APD) in rats and mice. *Toxicology*, **65**, 179–97

Eguchi, M., Yamaguchi, T., Shiota, E. and Handa, S. (1982). Fault of ossification and calcification and angular deformities of long bones in the mouse fetuses caused by high doses of ethane-1-hydroxy-1,1-diphosphonate (EHDP) during pregnancy. *Cong. Anom.*, **22**, 47–52

Flora, L., Hassing, G.S., Parfitt, A.M. and Villanueva, A.R. (1980). Comparative skeletal effects of two diphosphonates in dogs. *Metab. Bone Dis. Relat. Res.*, **2**, 389–407

Graepel, P., Bentley, P., Fritz, H., Miyamoto, M. and Slater, S.R. (1992). Reproduction toxicity studies with pamidronate. *Arzneim.-Forsch. Drug Res.*, **42**, 654–67

Nii, A., Fujimoto, R., Okazaki, A., Narita, K. and Miki, H. (1994). Intramembranous and endochondral bone changes induced by a new bisphosphonate (YM175) in the beagle dog. *Toxicol. Pathol.*, **22** (5), 536–44

Nixon, G.A., Buehler, E.V. and Newmann, E.A. (1972). Preliminary safety assessment of disodium etidronate as an additive to experimental oral hygiene products. *Toxicol. Appl. Pharmacol.*, **22**, 661–71

Nolen, G.A. and Buehler, E.V. (1971). The effects of disodium etidronate on the reproductive functions and embryogeny of albino rats and New Zealand rabbits. *Toxicol. Appl. Pharmacol.*, **18**, 548–61

Sakiyama, Y., Yamamoto, H., Soeda, Y., Tada, I., Oda, M., Nagasawa, S. and Ikeo, T. (1986). The effect of ethane-1-hydroxy-1,1-diphosphonate (EHDP) on fetal mice during pregnancy. Part 2: External anomalies. *J. Osaka Dent. Univ.*, **20**, 91–100

3. Bisphosphonates – clinical

3.1. INTRODUCTION

The clinical applications of bisphosphonates have focused on four areas. They are used as:

(a) Skeletal markers in the form of ^{99m}Tc derivatives for diagnostic purposes in nuclear medicine;

(b) Antiosteolytic agents in patients with increased bone destruction, especially Paget's disease, tumor bone disease and recently osteoporosis;

(c) Inhibitors of calcification in patients with ectopic calcification and ossification; and

(d) Antitartar agents added to toothpastes.

Only applications (b) and (c) are discussed in this book.

3.2. Paget's disease

3.2.1. Definition

Paget's disease is a localized and progressive disorder of bone remodeling and modeling, characterized by a focal increase in bone turnover. Originally called osteitis deformans, it was first described in 1876 by Sir James Paget.

3.2.2. Epidemiology

It is a fairly common disease, actually the second most common metabolic bone disease after osteoporosis in some countries. It has been estimated that in the countries where the ailment is prevalent, up to 5% of the population over the age of 50 is afflicted. The disease is frequent in Europe, with the exception of the Scandinavian countries, and is frequent in regions inhabited by European emigrants, such as North America and Australia. In contrast, it is rare in the Arab countries, as well as among blacks and Asians. It is almost always diagnosed in patients over the age of 40 and is probably somewhat more common in men than in women.

Paget's disease is fairly common and presents itself clinically after the age of 40.

3.2.3. Pathophysiology

For a yet unknown reason, bone turnover becomes abnormally increased at certain sites of the skeleton, with an increase in local remodeling and modeling. The cause is probably a slow paramyxovirus infection, in view of the presence of virus-like cellular inclusions in the osteoclasts, positive reactions with antisera raised against the measles virus, and the presence of mRNA of measles and other viruses in the cells. It has been suggested that in some cases the patients are infected by dogs afflicted by canine distemper. The initial event is a marked elevation of bone resorption, probably because of, among other reasons, an increase in IL-6 production by marrow and/or bone cells, leading to osteolytic lesions. A compensatory increase in formation occurs secondarily and induces an abnormally positive bone balance with sclerotic lesions and local deformations of the skeleton.

Coupling
p. 22

The disorder is due to localized foci of increased bone turnover following a local increase in resorption. The etiology is uncertain, possibly viral.

3.2.4. Clinical manifestations

Signs and symptoms

The condition is most commonly asymptomatic and is often discovered fortuitously during a routine measurement of serum alkaline phosphatase, an X-ray or more rarely a scintigraphic investigation. The lesions appear as lytic or sclerotic foci in the X-ray or as hot spots in the scintigraphy. The localization occurs mostly in the pelvis, the vertebrae, the scapulae, the larger long bones and the skull. They can be mono- or polyostotic. Sometimes a deformation of the bone, especially a bone enlargement, is present.

The disease is often asymptomatic and discovered during a routine measurement of serum alkaline phosphatase or an X-ray investigation.

Only approximately 5% of patients present symptoms. The most common complaint is pain, which may be very intense, and is most commonly secondary to a Pagetic localization in the back, the hip or a long bone. It can be caused by a microfracture, a fracture, or secondary joint disease. In the latter cases it will not respond to treatment, in contrast to the pain resulting from a Pagetic lesion itself.

Another complaint is bone deformity, especially bending of long bones and the spine, and enlargement of bones, such as the skull. The increase of the cranium has led to the term 'disease of the too small hat'. Deformities can lead to a variety of neurovascular symptoms, such as a vertebrobasilar artery syndrome and spinal cord dysfunction, due to compression of nerves and arteries. Deafness is common and is due to damage of the cochlear capsule. It is speculated that Paget's disease was the cause of Beethoven's deafness.

There can be an increase in vascularization in the afflicted bones which may lead to cardiac failure. Lastly, it must be remembered that some Pagetic lesions (about 1%) transform into an osteosarcoma, so that a close follow-up of all radiological changes is indicated.

> *Pain, bone deformities, fractures and neurovascular symptoms are commonly observed.*

Laboratory

Assessment of
turnover
p. 27

Laboratory findings reflect increased bone turnover, the indices of both bone formation and destruction being elevated. The elevation of bone formation is reflected in increased serum alkaline phosphatase, whereas serum osteocalcin (BGP) is, for unknown reasons, poorly correlated with the activity of the disease. Bone destruction is indicated by an increase in the fasting urinary hydroxyproline to creatinine ratio, and urinary pyridinoline crosslinks. There is a positive correlation between the extension of the disease and the biochemical markers. In monostotic disease they can therefore be normal. The markers are also used for evaluation of the effect of treatment and the detection of a relapse.

> *Useful chemical investigations are serum alkaline phosphatase, fasting urinary hydroxyproline and urinary pyridinoline crosslinks.*

X-ray pictures show, besides osseous deformations and enlargement of the size of certain bones, local areas of increased bone density, an accentuated trabecular pattern and sclerotic changes. These can be so accentuated that they lead to the so-called ivory vertebrae, which are sometimes difficult to distinguish from metastases.

Of great diagnostic use is scintigraphy with pertechnetate-labeled compounds where the lesions show up as hot spots. It is the best method for establishing the map of the pagetic sites in the patient.

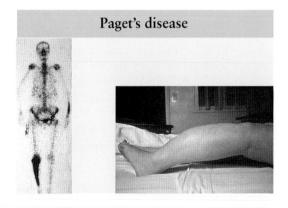

Paget's disease

Fig. 3.2-1 ^{99m}Tc-labeled bisphosphonate scintigram of a patient with Paget's disease. Intense hot spots are seen in the tibia, which is deformed. (Courtesy of Drs P.J. Meunier and P.D. Delmas.)

Useful radiophysical investigations are radiography and scintigraphy.

The histology of Pagetic bone is characterized by the signs of an extremely rapid turnover. The lesions comprise a mosaic structure of areas of resorption, with a large number of osteoclasts, and of formation sites. Characteristically the new bone is not lamellar but woven, which explains its brittleness despite the osteosclerosis.

Woven bone
p. 11

→ Fig. 3.2-2 Histology of Pagetic bone. Left: Picture of high bone turnover with many osteoclasts. Right: New bone of woven type. (Courtesy of Dr P.J. Meunier.)

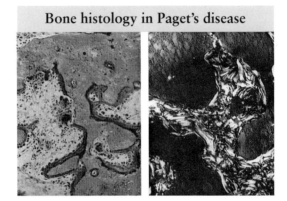

Bone histology in Paget's disease

Diagnosis

The diagnosis of Paget's disease is made by radiography, scintigraphy, the laboratory evaluation of bone turnover and the clinical picture.

Follow-up of evolution

The evolution of the disease is followed by assessing the symptoms, the biochemical indices of bone turnover and scintigraphy, the latter being
→ used more rarely. From the indices of bone formation, serum alkaline phosphatase is more reliable than osteocalcin in this disease. For assessing bone resorption, both urinary hydroxyproline and pyridinoline crosslinks are excellent. Most often it is sufficient to follow only one parameter, the least expensive one being serum alkaline phosphatase.

Assessment
of turnover
pp. 27–28

Indices of bone turnover
Formation
Serum alkaline phosphatase
Resorption
Urinary hydroxyproline Urinary pyridinoline crosslinks

Fig. 3.2-3   Bone turnover indices used to monitor treatment in Paget's disease.

The evolution of the disease and its treatment are usually monitored by following one of the biochemical indices of bone turnover. The least expensive and most used is serum alkaline phosphatase.

3.2.5.   Treatment with drugs other than bisphosphonates

Treatment should be offered to all symptomatic patients as well as to asymptomatic patients with involvement of skeletal areas that have a potential to give rise to complications, such as the skull, vertebral bodies, long bones and near major joints. However, many patients, especially those in whom diagnosis was fortuitous and who have no symptoms, need no treatment.

Practically the only treatment, apart from bisphosphonates, is calcitonin. This hormone can be effective in decreasing bone turnover in Pagetic patients and in improving clinical signs and symptoms. Calcitonin has, however, some drawbacks in comparison with bisphosphonates. Bone turnover relapses occur earlier and are more frequent after discontinuation of treatment, and sometimes even during therapy. In addition, some patients show unpleasant adverse reactions, such as vascular symptoms.

Plicamycin has been practically abandoned because of its toxicity.

The only treatment other than bisphosphonates is calcitonin.

3.2.6. Treatment with bisphosphonates

Preclinical studies

No animal model exists for Paget's disease. However, results obtained in animals with normal or experimentally increased bone resorption have proven to be good predictors of the effect in humans.

Inhibition of bone resorption pp. 38–45

Clinical studies

The bisphosphonates are developing as the therapy of choice in Paget's disease. All bisphosphonates that have been tested so far have proven to be active in decreasing bone turnover. The difference between the compounds lies in their potency and in their adverse event profile. They are all focally concentrated in the involved areas because of the high local bone turnover. This is probably a major cause of their long-lasting effect.

Effects

Most clinical studies in Paget's disease deal with etidronate, pamidronate and clodronate. Other bisphosphonates showing clinical efficacy include alendronate, neridronate, olpadronate, risedronate, tiludronate and zoledronate. The effects observed are quantitatively very similar, but differ with respect to the rapidity with which they develop and the total amount of decrease in turnover obtained.

Chemical structures pp. 35–36

The effects of the various bisphosphonates are qualitatively similar, the differences lying in their potency and adverse event profile.

The largest number of investigations has been performed with etidronate, the first bisphosphonate to be used in this disease, followed by pamidronate. The initial report, which was also the first report in which an effect of a bisphosphonate on bone resorption in a human was demonstrated, dates back to 1971. Both bone resorption and formation were decreased. This action on bone turnover has been well documented in numerous subsequent studies (*see* Fig. 3.2-4).

→ The effect on resorption precedes that on formation, suggesting that, as in animals, the decrease in formation is secondary, due to the coupling between the two processes. This time lapse has the practical consequence that urinary hydroxyproline is a better marker to assess the acute effect of treatment than alkaline phosphatase. The latter will give useful information only after about 4 weeks, and often longer (*see* Fig 3.2-5).

Coupling p. 22

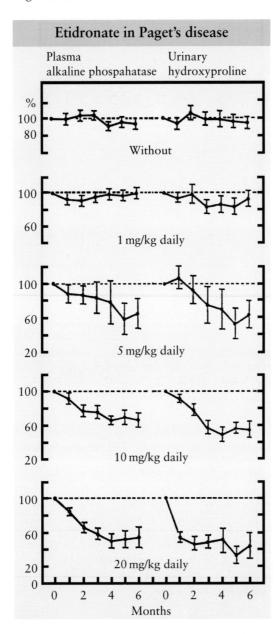

Fig. 3.2-4 Effect of various doses of etidronate on the indices of bone resorption and bone formation in Paget's disease, expressed in percentage of initial values. (Adapted from Russell, R.G.G. *et al.* (1974). *Lancet*, **1**, 894–8. Reproduced with permission from the author and the publisher.)

→ Fig. 3.2-5 Effect of 300 mg/day of clodronate given intravenously for 5 days on bone turnover. Note that bone resorption (urinary hydroxyproline) decreases before bone formation (alkaline phosphatase). (Adapted from Kanis, J.A. and McCloskey, E.V. (1990). Reproduced from Kanis, J.A. (ed.) *Calcium Metabolism. Progress in Basic and Clinical Pharmacology*, vol. 4, pp. 89–136, with copyright permission from the author and S. Karger AG, Basel.)

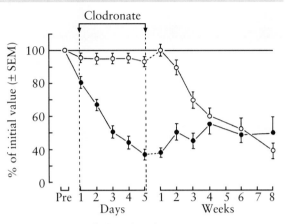

Bisphosphonates decrease both bone resorption and bone formation. The effect on formation occurs somewhat later and is probably secondary to the physiological coupling between the two processes

The decrease in bone turnover can be accompanied by a small decrease in serum of ionized calcium and of phosphate, and an elevation of serum PTH and $1,25(OH)_2$ vitamin D. The latter are often seen when patients with a high level of osteolysis are treated with a powerful inhibitor of bone resorption. In order to avoid the increase in PTH, some advise administration of the bisphosphonates, especially in patients with severe disease, together with 0.5–1.0 g calcium. Sometimes, 400–800 units of vitamin D per day are also used. In contrast to other bisphosphonates, and for an unknown reason, etidronate increases plasma phosphate, as is also the case with this bisphosphonate in other indications.

Morphological studies also indicate a decrease in turnover. The number of osteoclasts is diminished, but the virus-like cellular inclusions in the nuclei and the measles-type viral antigens in the osteoclasts persist unmodified. It is interesting that the bone formed under treatment with bisphosphonates returns to a lamellar organization, in contrast to the woven bone formation typical of this disease.

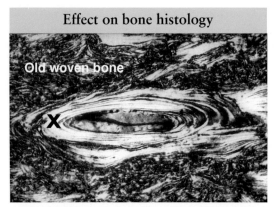

Effect on bone histology

Old woven bone

X

Fig 3.2-6 Effect of etidronate (above) and clodronate (below) on bone histology in Paget's disease. The new bone formed is now lamellar (X), with no more bone woven, either in the cortex (above) or in the trabeculae (below). (Courtesy of Dr P.J. Meunier. Reproduced from Meunier, P.J. *et al.* (1987). *Am. J. Med.*, **82** (Suppl. 2A), 71–8, with permission from the author and publisher.)

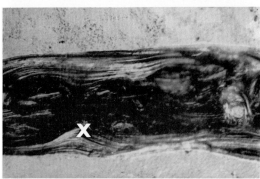

X

Bisphosphonates improve the morphology of bone. The number of osteoclasts is decreased, and the new bone formed is lamellar instead of woven.

Bone pain usually decreases, except when it is due to arthritic changes. It can, however, sometimes be increased with etidronate, and occasionally with other bisphosphonates. In the case of etidronate the dosage is likely to be too high and should be reduced. With aminobisphosphonates, the pain occurs earlier, within the first days, and may be related to the acute-phase-like syndrome often observed with these compounds. It resolves spontaneously and does not require reduction of the dose.

Bone pain is usually decreased. If it is increased with etidronate, the dose of the bisphosphonate is likely to be too high.

The finding that bone deformities, for example in the face, as well as neurological spinal syndromes can be improved, suggests that treatment not only stops the progression of the disease, but can also lead to an amelioration of pre-existing lesions. Elevated cardiac output is brought back to normal. Lastly, treatment with bisphosphonates markedly improves the pathological uptake of radioactive technetium. Radiologically, although major changes are mostly not striking, the refilling of the V-shaped lesions of long bones or of osteoporosis circumscripta of the skull is not uncommon.

Neurological spinal syndromes as well as scintigraphic scans of the skeleton and certain radiological alterations are improved.

The decrease in bone turnover, as well as the other improvements, can last for a long time after the discontinuation of treatment, often years. Some patients have actually not relapsed for up to 12 years. This is much less so in the case of calcitonin treatment.

The therapeutic effect on bone turnover can last for a long time, often years, after treatment has been discontinued.

Treatment regimens

Dosage has often been calculated in Paget's disease, as well as in other disorders, according to body weight. This is only meaningful if the latter gives a good reflection of the weight of the skeleton, which is true in children, but most often not in adults. Adjusting the dose according to the fat content of the body has no scientific rationale. If a correction is to be made, which is in general not useful, it would be better to take as a basis the ideal weight of the patient.

Prescribing a dose per kg of body weight is in most cases not useful in the adult.

The effect of treatment is monitored, as mentioned above, by one of the biochemical parameters of bone turnover, serum alkaline phosphatase being today the simplest and least expensive. In the future crosslinks may become increasingly used. It must, however, be remembered that the indices of bone formation respond later than those of bone resorption. The aim of the treatment is to decrease bone turnover to the normal range. Indeed, a relationship appears to exist between the decrease in turnover obtained during treatment and the duration of the effect. If this is not possible with a specific bisphosphonate, even after longer therapy, a more potent compound should be used if available. The plateau is usually reached within 3–6 months for alkaline phosphatase,

Effect on turnover p. 75

faster for the parameters of bone resorption. Treatment is then discontinued until the indices of bone turnover start to increase again. At what elevation one should start to resume treatment is difficult to stipulate. An increase of 25% has been suggested.

> *Treatment should aim to normalize turnover, as assessed by one of the biochemical markers, e.g. alkaline phosphatase. This occurs usually within 6 months. Treatment is resumed when the biochemical markers rise again by at least 25%.*

Recent results show that, as in tumor bone disease, patients with more active forms of the disease require higher total amounts of bisphosphonates. One explanation is that the bisphosphonate administered is distributed into more areas of high turnover, so that the amount deposited in each focal lesion is smaller.

> *Patients with more severe disease require higher amounts of bisphosphonates.*

Alendronate

Oral administration of 40 mg daily for 6 months induced a decrease of about 70–80% in bone turnover, approximately 40–65% of the patients reaching normal levels.

> *A dose of 40 mg daily per os of alendronate normalizes the turnover in about half the patients.*

Clodronate

Oral daily doses between 400 and 1600 mg can normalize biochemical parameters, 800 mg administered for 3–6 months being apparently sufficient for maximal effect. At this dose, 40% of the patients normalize their turnover. Treatment for 1 month is as effective as treatment for 6 months, but the duration of the effect appears to be shorter. It is also possible to give 300 mg daily for 5 days as an intravenous infusion.

> *A dose of 800 mg daily per os for 3 months, or 300 mg daily intravenously for 5 days is usually a sufficient regimen for maximal effect.*

Etidronate

The dose of etidronate necessary to inhibit bone resorption in patients with Paget's disease is, as in the animal, not too different from that inhibiting normal bone mineralization. Since intestinal absorption is variable between patients, and even within the same person, the optimal dosage is sometimes difficult to establish. The currently recommended daily dose of etidronate is 5 mg/kg daily orally, which corresponds usually to 400 mg, for no longer than 6 months. It is effective in decreasing bone turnover substantially and is usually very well tolerated, although not always devoid of mineralization impairment. However, about 70% of the patients do not normalize turnover at this regimen. If this is the case, or if resistance develops during a later course of therapy, as is the case in many patients, higher doses, such as 10 mg/kg, have been proposed. However, the drawback here is the danger of inhibition of mineralization. Despite the fact that this defect will heal relatively quickly, probably within months, when the treatment is stopped, it is preferable to switch to a more powerful bisphosphonate, if available. Another possibility suggested by some is the intravenous infusion of 300–600 mg daily for 5 days.

In general after completion of a course of treatment, a second course should not be started before 3 months, preferably longer.

Effect on turnover p. 74

Intestinal absorption p. 57

Inhibition of mineralization pp. 148–149

The dosage recommendation for etidronate is difficult, since the active dose required in some patients is near that inducing osteomalacia. The most commonly used dose of etidronate is 400 mg/day orally for not longer than 6 months. However, the majority of patients do not normalize their turnover at this dose and may develop resistance after a few courses.

Etidronate is widely available for the treatment of Paget's disease.

Commercially available bisphosphonates pp. 157–170

Olpadronate

The daily administration of 200 mg orally or of 4 mg intravenously of this newer bisphosphonate for 10 days or longer resulted in excellent results with a recurrence-free period of over 2 years.

Olpadronate given at 200 mg orally or 4 mg intravenously for 10 days gives good results.

Pamidronate

Commercially
available
bisphosphonates
pp. 157–170

Pamidronate has recently been introduced in various countries for use in Paget's disease. Of the three commercially available bisphosphonates, it is the most potent. Many different regimens have been used in the past, and it is difficult to draw precise, well founded conclusions as to the optimal one. One infusion of 60 mg was found sufficient to normalize the biochemical parameters of turnover in about one-half of the patients afflicted by a mild form of the disease and to induce a long-lasting effect. To normalize more patients, and in more severe cases, higher doses are required. In all instances the producer proposes intermittent infusions of either 30 mg weekly or 60 mg every 2 weeks for a duration of 6 weeks, which corresponds to a total dose of 180 mg. Such a treatment normalizes the turnover in up to 90% of the patients with mild to moderate disease and between 25% and 66% in patients with severe disease. Treatment can be repeated after an interval of 6 months. The compound must always be dissolved in 250 ml for up to 60 mg and in 500 ml for up to 90 mg and be infused not faster than in 1 hour and 2 hours, respectively.

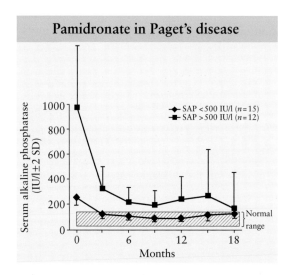

Fig. 3.2-7 Effect of 180 mg intravenously of pamidronate given by infusions of 30 mg once a week for 6 weeks in patients with mild to moderate and severe Paget's disease. SAP, serum alkaline phosphatase. (Based on patients reported in Richardson, D.C. *et al.* (1990). *Calcium Reg. Bone Metab.*, **10**, 509–14. Reproduced with permission from the author.)

Adverse effects
p. 151

Successful regimens also include 250 mg or more orally for 6 months, lower doses being less effective. However, in view of gastrointestinal adverse events, parenteral administration is clearly preferred. Furthermore pamidronate is commercially available in an oral form in only very few countries.

Pamidronate is very effective in decreasing bone turnover. In view of the gastrointestinal disturbances at high doses, the intravenous route is usually used today. While one infusion of 60 mg is sufficient in mild cases, higher total doses, usually 180 mg given in several infusions, are required in more severe ones.

Today pamidronate is registered for Paget's disease in a few countries. It is, however, foreseen to make the intravenous form more widely available soon.

Commercially available bisphosphonates pp. 157–170

Risedronate

A dose of 30 mg given orally daily for 12 weeks to patients with severe disease, followed if necessary by a second treatment after a 16-week interval, normalized alkaline phosphatase in about half the patients.

Tiludronate

Previously the active oral doses of tiludronate ranged between 400 and 800 mg/day orally given for 3 months, 800 mg being considered optimal.

Tiludronate in Paget's disease

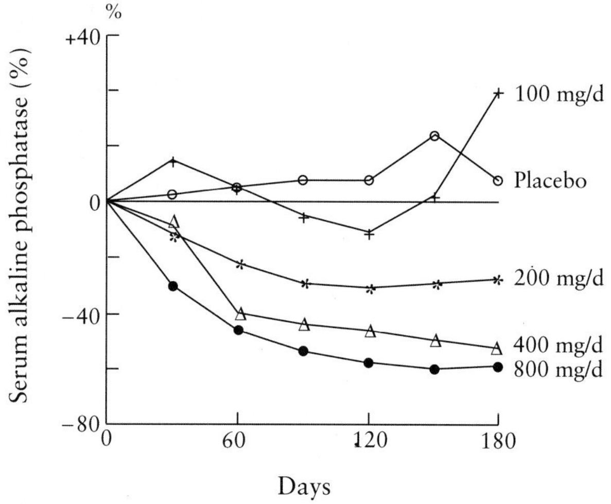

Fig. 3.2-8 Effect of tiludronate former formulation given orally for 3 months on bone turnover in Paget's disease. (Adapted from Reginster, J.Y. *et al.* (1992). Reproduced from *Arthritis Rheum.*, 35, 967–74, with copyright permission from the author and J.B. Lippincott Company, Philadelphia, PA.)

Paget's disease

Higher doses, such as 1200 mg, were accompanied by gastrointestinal side effects. Today, with a new formulation, the daily oral administration of 400 mg for 3–6 months was found as effective as 800 mg of the previous formulation. This dose normalizes the biochemical parameters in 25–40% of the patients.

> *Oral doses of 400 mg/day of tiludronate given for 3 months are also effective.*

Other bisphosphonates

Recently ibandronate given in a single intravenous dose of 2 mg and zoledronate given in a single intravenous dose of 0.4 mg have also been shown to be very active.

Chemical
structures
pp. 35–36

> *Alendronate, ibandronate, olpadronate, risedronate and zoledronate are all active at very low doses.*

Conclusion

> *Today bisphosphonates are the drugs of choice in Paget's disease. Etidronate is commercially available in most countries. In the countries where the more potent alendronate, clodronate, olpadronate, pamidronate, or tiludronate are or will be available, they are excellent alternatives.*

Recommended selected reading

Paget's disease

Books

Kanis, J.A. (1991). *Pathophysiology and Treatment of Paget's Disease of Bone*. (London: Martin Dunitz)

Reviews

Altman, R.D. (1992). Paget's disease of bone. In Coe, F.L. and Favus, M.J. (eds.) *Disorders of Bone and Mineral Metabolism*, pp. 1027–64. (New York: Raven Press)

Anderson, D.C. (1993). Paget's disease. In Mundy, G.R. and Martin, T.J. (eds.) *Physiology and Pharmacology of Bone. Handbook of Experimental Pharmacology*, vol. 107, pp. 419–41. (Berlin, Heidelberg, New York: Springer Verlag)

Hosking, D.J. (1990). Advances in the management of Paget's disease of bone. *Drugs*, 40, 829–40

Siris, E.S. (1990). Paget's disease of bone. In Favus, M.J. (ed.) *Primer on the Metabolic Bone Diseases and Disorders of Mineral Metabolism*, pp. 253–9. (Kelseyville, CA: American Society for Bone and Mineral Research)

Bisphosphonates

Reviews

Kanis, J.A. (1991). Drugs used for the treatment of Paget's disease. In Kanis, J.A. (ed.) *Pathophysiology and Treatment of Paget's Disease of Bone*, pp. 159–216. (London: Martin Dunitz)

Alendronate

Original articles

O'Doherty, D.P., Bickerstaff, D.R., McCloskey, E.V., Hamdy, N.A.T., Beneton, M.N.C., Harris, S., Mian, M. and Kanis, J.A. (1990). Treatment of Paget's disease of bone with aminohydroxybutylidene bisphosphonate. *J. Bone Miner. Res.*, 5, 483–91

Clodronate

Reviews

Kanis, J.A. and McCloskey, E.V. (1990). The use of clodronate in disorders of calcium and skeletal metabolism. In Kanis, J.A. (ed.) *Calcium Metabolism. Progress in Basic and Clinical Pharmacology*, vol. 4, pp. 89–136. (Basel: Karger)

Plosker, G.L. and Goa, K.L. (1994). Clodronate. A review of its pharmacological properties and therapeutic efficacy in resorptive bone disease. *Drugs*, 47, 945–82

Original articles

Delmas, P.D., Chapuy, M.C., Vignon, E., Charhon, S., Briançon, D., Alexandre, C., Edouard, C. and Meunier, P.J. (1982). Long term effects of dichloromethylene diphosphonate in Paget's disease of bone. *J. Clin. Endocrinol. Metab.*, 54, 837–44

Douglas, D.L., Duckworth, T., Kanis, J.A., Preston, C., Beard, D.J., Smith, T.W.D., Underwood, I., Woodhead, J.S. and Russell, R.G.G. (1980). Biochemical and clinical responses to dichloromethylene diphosphonate (Cl_2MDP) in Paget's disease of bone. *Arthritis Rheum.*, 23, 1185–92

Yates, A.J.P., Percival, R.C., Gray, R.E.S., Atkins, R.M., Urwin, G.H., Hamdy, N.A.T., Preston, C.J., Beneton, M.N.C., Russell, R.G.G. and Kanis, J.A. (1985). Intravenous clodronate in the treatment and retreatment of Paget's disease of bone. *Lancet*, 1, 1474–7

Paget's disease

Etidronate

Reviews

Dunn, C.J., Fitton, A. and Sorkin, E.M. (1994). Etidronic acid. A review of its pharmacological properties and therapeutic efficacy in resorptive bone disease. *Drugs Aging*, 5, 446–74

Original articles

Altman, R.D., Johnston, C.C., Khairi, M.R.A., Wellman, H., Serafini, A.N. and Sankey, R.R. (1973). Influence of disodium etidronate on clinical and laboratory manifestations of Paget's disease of bone (osteitis deformans). *N. Engl. J. Med.*, 289, 1379–84

Boyce, B.F., Smith, L., Fogelman, I., Johnston, E., Ralston, S. and Boyle, I.T. (1984). Focal osteomalacia due to low-dose diphosphonate therapy in Paget's disease. *Lancet*, 1, 821–4

de Vries, H.R. and Bijvoet, O.L.M. (1974). Results of prolonged treatment of Paget's disease of bone with disodium ethane-1-hydroxy-1,1-diphosphonate (EHDP). *Neth. J. Med.*, 17, 281–98

Nagant de Deuxchaisnes, C., Rombouts-Lindemans, C., Huaux, J.P., Devogelaer, J.P., Malghem, J. and Maldague, B. (1979). Roentgenologic evaluation of the action of the diphosphonate EHDP and of combined therapy (EHDP and calcitonin) in Paget's disease of bone. *Mol. Endocrinol.*, 1, 405–33

Russell, R.G.G., Smith, R., Preston, C., Walton, R.J. and Woods, C.G. (1974). Diphosphonates in Paget's disease. *Lancet*, 1 894–8

Smith, R., Russell, R.G.G. and Bishop, M. (1971). Diphosphonates and Paget's disease of bone. *Lancet*, 1, 945–7

Pamidronate

Reviews

Fitton, A. and McTavish, D. (1991) Pamidronate: a review of its pharmacological properties and therapeutic efficacy in resorptive bone disease. *Drugs*, 41, 289–318

Original articles

Frijlink, W.B., Bijvoet, O.L.M., te Velde, J. and Heynen, G. (1979). Treatment of Paget's disease with (3-amino-1-hydroxypropylidene)-1,1-bisphosphonate (A.P.D.). *Lancet*, 1, 799–803

Gallacher, S.J., Boyce, B.F., Patel, U., Jenkins, A., Ralston, S.H. and Boyle, I.T. (1991). Clinical experience with pamidronate in the treatment of Paget's disease of bone. *Ann. Rheum. Dis.*, 50, 930–3

Ryan, P.J., Sherry, M., Gibson, T. and Fogelman, I. (1991) Treatment of Paget's disease by weekly infusions of 3-aminohydroxypropylidene-1,1-bisphosphonate (APD). *Br. J. Rheumatol.*, 31, 97–101

Thiébaud, D., Jaeger, P., Gobelet, C., Jacquet, A.F. and Burckhardt, P. (1988). Single infusion of the bisphosphonate AHPrBP (APD) as treatment of Paget's disease of bone. *Am. J. Med.*, 85, 207–12

Tiludronate

Reviews

Reginster, J.Y.L. (1992). Oral tiludronate: pharmacological properties and potential use-fulness in Paget's disease of bone and osteoporosis. *Bone*, 13, 351–4

Original articles

Audran, M., Clochon, P., Ethgen, D., Mazières, B. and Renier, J.C. (1989). Treatment of Paget's disease of bone with (4-chloro-phenyl)thiomethylene bisphosphonate. *Clin. Rheumatol.*, 8, 71–9

Reginster, J.Y., Colson, F., Morlock, G., Combe, B., Ethgen, D. and Geusens, P. (1992). Evaluation of the efficacy and safety of oral tiludronate in Paget's disease of bone. A double-blind, multiple-dosage, placebo-controlled study. *Arthritis Rheum.*, 35, 967–74

Reginster, J.Y., Treves, R., Renier, J.C., Amor, B., Sany, J., Ethgen, D., Picot, C. and Franchimont, P. (1994). Efficacy and tolerability of a new formulation of oral tilu-dronate (tablet) in the treatment of Paget's disease of bone. *J. Bone Miner. Res.*, 9, 615–19

Other bisphosphonates

Original articles

Atkins, R.M., Yates, A.J.P., Gray, R.E.S., Urwin, G.H., Hamdy, N.A.T., Beneton, M.N.C., Rosini, S. and Kanis, J.A. (1987). Aminohexane diphosphonate in the treatment of Paget's disease of bone. *J. Bone Miner. Res.*, 2, 273–9

Delmas, P.D., Chapuy, M.C., Edouard, C. and Meunier, P.J. (1987). Beneficial effects of aminohexane diphosphonate in patients with Paget's disease of bone resistant to sodium etidronate. *Am. J. Med.*, 83, 276–82

Schweitzer, D.H., Zwinderman, A.H., Vermeij, P., Bijvoet, O.L.M. and Papapoulos, S.E. (1993). Improved treatment of Paget's disease with dimethylaminohydroxypropylidene bisphosphonate. *J. Bone Miner. Res.*, 8, 175–82

3.3. OSTEOLYTIC TUMOR BONE DISEASE

3.3.1. Definition

This is a condition in which tumors of various origins induce bone destruction, either through local invasion, or at a distance by secreting bone-resorbing products into the bloodstream.

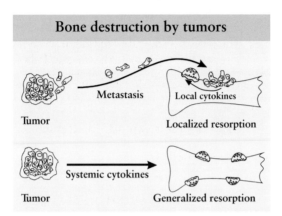

Fig. 3.3-1 Mechanisms of malignant bone destruction.

3.3.2. Pathophysiology

Bone
resorption
p. 19

Local erosion is seen mostly in metastases of carcinoma of the breast and lung and in hematological malignancies, especially multiple myeloma. Breast cancer is frequently associated with bone metastases, 90% of patients who died of this disease having such metastases. The mechanism of resorption of bone is not well elucidated. It appears that tumor cells can secrete a series of bone-resorbing cytokines such as the recently identified PTH-related peptide, TGFα, TNFα, TNFβ, M-CSF, interleukins, prostaglandins and others, which will induce locally osteoclast-mediated bone resorption. It is possible that certain tumor cells themselves can also destroy bone.

Generalized bone destruction is seen among other conditions in carcinoma of the lung, breast, head and neck, kidney and ovary. Bone resorption is induced via the systemic production of osteolytic factors, especially PTH-related peptide, by a tumor localized elsewhere in the body. If the condition is accompanied by hypercalcemia, it is called 'humoral hypercalcemia of malignancy (HHM)'. Both mechanisms can be operating simultaneously.

Tumors can induce bone resorption either locally when present in the bone, or by the systemic secretion of osteolytic factors when localized outside the skeleton (humoral hypercalcemia of malignancy).

The localized bone resorption leads to pathological fractures and pain, which are the most common features of tumor bone disease. Another consequence is hypercalcemia, cancer being the most common cause of this disturbance when clinically significant. The tumors most frequently associated with hypercalcemia are carcinoma of the breast, the lung and upper respiratory tract, myeloma and lymphomas. About a quarter of patients with breast cancer develop hypercalcemia, and about a quarter of patients with malignant hypercalcemia have carcinoma of the breast.

Fig. 3.3-2 Tumors that induce hypercalcemia of malignancy most frequently.

Tumors inducing hypercalcemia

- Breast
- Respiratory tract
- Myeloma and lymphomas
- Kidney

A consequence of tumors, especially cancer of the breast and lung, and myeloma, is hypercalcemia.

The mechanisms inducing hypercalcemia are complex, the increase in blood calcium not being due to bone lysis alone. Three main mechanisms are involved:

(1) Increased bone destruction, either local or generalized, which brings about a release of calcium from the skeleton and consequently an increase in the flow of calcium through the extracellular space. This mechanism appears to be the main cause of hypercalcemia in patients with hematological malignancies such as myeloma and in many patients with metastases;

Calcium homeostasis pp. 23–26

(2) Increased tubular reabsorption of calcium in the kidney, as a result of factors produced by tumor cells, probably mostly PTH-related peptide. This peptide, which is also produced by certain non-tumor tissues and probably plays its main role in fetal life, has a sequence that resembles parathyroid hormone and acts on the same receptor. The renal mechanism is seen in solid tumors such as squamous cell carcinoma of

the lung and of other organs. In many solid tumors with bone metastases both the osseous and renal mechanisms can coexist;

(3) Volume depletion, inducing hypercalcemia by various mechanisms. It increases blood calcium by hemoconcentration and by enhancing proximal tubular reabsorption of calcium. Tumor disease is often accompanied by dehydration, which can be very extensive and lead to renal failure. The dehydration is due in part to an increase in sodium excretion induced by the hypercalcemia. Furthermore the decrease in glomerular filtration can lead to an impairment of calcium excretion. Therefore, rehydration is always the first therapeutic step in cases of threatening hypercalcemia, and it is very often followed by a drop in calcemia occurring without any other treatment.

(4) Less frequent mechanisms include, as in myeloma, a decrease in bone formation, which can contribute to hypercalcemia through the diminished efflux of calcium from the extracellular space to bone. In some lymphomas, intestinal absorption of calcium is increased due to elevated $1, 25(OH)_2$ vitamin D, which can also contribute to the hypercalcemia.

Calcium homeostasis pp. 23–26

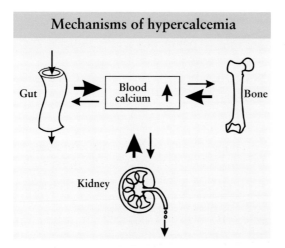

Fig. 3.3-3 Mechanisms of hypercalcemia in tumor bone disease.

Hypercalcemia in tumor bone disease is caused essentially by increased osteolysis, increased renal reabsorption of calcium and dehydration.

The fact that hypercalcemia is produced by various mechanisms has therapeutic consequences. Since only bone resorption is influenced by bisphosphonates, calcemia will be less influenced by these compounds in patients where non-osteolytic mechanisms are prominent. This is the case, for example, in humoral hypercalcemia of malignancy. In contrast, hypercalciuria, which is increased in most cases as a consequence of elevated bone resorption only, will be corrected effectively in nearly all cases.

Bisphosphonates most effectively correct hypercalcemia due to osteolytic tumors located in bone and producing no circulating cytokines. They are less effective in hypercalcemia caused by circulating factors, especially from tumors outside the skeleton, which also affect other organs, especially the kidney.

3.3.3. Clinical manifestations

Signs and symptoms

The clinical manifestations are those of tumor osteolysis, namely pain and fractures, and of hypercalcemia and its multiple metabolic consequences.

Fig. 3.3-4 Main clinical manifestations in tumor bone disease.

Tumor bone disease

- Pain
- Fractures
- Hypercalcemia syndrome

→   Symptoms of hypercalcemia appear mainly in the neurological, gastrointestinal, cardiovascular and renal systems. In some cases, the hypercalcemia can lead to a life-threatening condition which must be dealt with immediately (*see* Fig. 3.3-5).

The other symptoms are those of the underlying tumor disease.

The main clinical manifestations of tumor osteolysis are pain, fractures and the hypercalcemic syndrome. Sometimes life-threatening hypercalcemic crises may occur.

Laboratory

The main biochemical investigations useful in osteolytic bone disease are serum calcium and urinary excretion of calcium, hydroxyproline and

Assessment of resorption p. 27

Signs and symptoms of hypercalcemia	
• Psychiatric	Unspecific
• Neurological	Drowsiness, lethargy
• Gastrointestinal	Constipation, vomiting, anorexia
• Cardiovascular	ECG changes, arrhythmias
• Renal	Hyposthenuria, nephro-calcinosis, renal failure
• Hypercalcemic crisis	

Fig. 3.3-5 Clinical features of the hyper-calcemic syndrome. ←

pyridinoline crosslinks. If lesions with bone formation are present, such as in metastases of prostate and sometimes of breast carcinoma, measurement of serum alkaline phosphatase or preferably bone-specific alkaline phosphatase, to distinguish from changes due to liver metastases, is helpful. It should be remembered that ionized calcium, which is the ← physiologically relevant form, can be underestimated in the presence of the hypoalbuminemia which influences the relative distribution between ionized and bound calcium, and which is often present in cancer patients. A simple correction factor is to add to the measured total calcium 0.08 mg/100 ml for each gram of albumin lower than 40 g/l.

The radiophysical examinations used are mainly X-rays, scintigraphy, computer tomography and, more recently, magnetic resonance imaging, which is extremely sensitive.

The main biochemical investigations of skeletal disturbances are measurement of serum calcium and alkaline phosphatase, as well as urinary excretion of calcium, hydroxyproline and pyridinoline crosslinks. The radiophysical techniques used are X-rays, scintigraphy, computer tomography and magnetic resonance imaging.

Diagnosis

The diagnosis of skeletal involvement is made from the clinical symptoms, by radiographic and scintigraphic skeletal investigations and by the measurement of blood calcium and the biochemical parameters of bone resorption.

Follow-up of evolution

The parameters followed are mostly blood calcium and in certain cases alkaline phosphatase, urinary excretion of calcium and sometimes hydroxyproline or pyridinoline crosslinks, as well as pain, fractures and the radiological evolution of osteolytic foci. The most frequent investigation is of calcemia, which is easy to perform. Futhermore, hypercalcemia is one of the disturbances in tumor-induced bone disease with the most severe clinical consequences and which, therefore, has to be treated.

Fig. 3.3-6 Parameters most often monitored during treatment.

Main investigations

- Serum calcium
- Urinary calcium
- Pain
- Fractures
- Osteolytic foci

The parameters usually followed during the treatment of tumor bone disease are most of all calcemia, urinary calcium, pain, fractures and osteolytic foci.

3.3.4. Treatment with drugs other than bisphosphonates

Up to now, the main treatment of osseous involvement besides excision of the primary tumor, chemo- or radiotherapy, has been plicamycin (mythramycin), an inhibitor of RNA synthesis. However, because of its toxicity, especially in the liver, bone marrow and kidney, it is only infrequently used today.

Hypercalcemia in the acute stage is first treated with fluid expansion. Volume repletion (2–4 l over the initial 24–48 h) is the first therapy when dehydration is present. However, care must be taken to avoid overhydration. Other interventions are less efficacious. Calcitonin, possibly associated with glucocorticoids, has sometimes been given in both acute and chronic hypercalcemia. The use of loop diuretics, such as furosemide, is of uncertain efficacy in decreasing blood calcium and may lead to a serious disturbance of fluid and electrolyte balance.

In view of this unsatisfactory situation, the bisphosphonates have become today the drugs of choice.

3.3.5. Treatment with bisphosphonates

Preclinical studies

In organ culture, bisphosphonates added to the culture medium inhibit the resorption of mouse calvaria induced by supernatants of breast or other cancer cells.

In vivo, bisphosphonates normalize or prevent the increased calciuria ← induced in rats by subcutaneous implantation of various tumor cells. In contrast they do not always entirely prevent or correct hypercalcemia. The cause of this discrepancy is, as discussed above, due to the fact that in some of these models, hypercalcemia is induced by the systemic production of PTH-related peptide, which increases not only bone resorption but also tubular reabsorption of calcium, on which bisphosphonates are inactive.

Mechanism of hyper-calcemia pp. 87–89

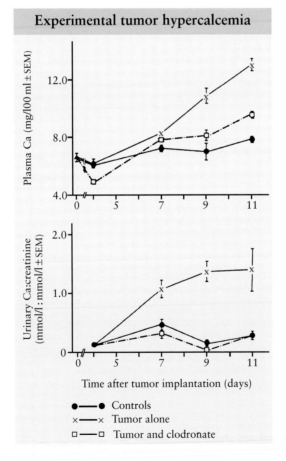

Fig. 3.3-7 Effect of clodronate administered daily on tumoral hyper-calcemia and hyper-calciuria in the rat implanted subcutaneously with Walker carcinosar-coma cells. (Adapted from Rizzoli, R. and Fleisch, H. (1987). *Calcif. Tissue Int.*, **41**, 202–7, with copyright permission from the authors and Springer-Verlag, Heidelberg.)

Bisphosphonates prevent hypercalcemia partially, and prevent hypercalciuria completely, in rats implanted subcutaneously with tumor cells.

Bisphosphonates also prevent or slow down bone resorption due to actual tumor invasion. Thus, etidronate, clodronate and pamidronate all decrease bone destruction induced by Walker carcinosarcoma cells injected into the iliac artery of the rat, a procedure whereby the cells are seeded into the bone. Risedronate decreases the development of bone metastases after intracardiac inoculation of tumor cells. Bisphosphonates are also effective when various tumor cell types are directly implanted into the bone or in the vicinity of the bone.

Bisphosphonates inhibit local bone destruction by tumors.

In contrast, bisphosphonates have no effect on the development of the various tumors in soft tissues. Thus, they do not inhibit the multiplication of tumor cells and are therefore not active on the tumor itself, but exert their action only by inhibiting the osteolytic process. As a secondary consequence this will, however, induce an inhibition of osseous tumor invasion, possibly in part by a decrease of local cytokines released when bone is resorbed, and which may stimulate replication of cancer cells.

The bisphosphonates do not directly inhibit the growth of the tumoral tissue.

Recently methotrexate–bisphosphonate conjugates have been synthesized and found to be active in the rat Walker carcinosarcoma model. Using bisphosphonates to bring chemostatic agents to the skeleton is an interesting new procedure.

Binding chemostatic agents to bisphosphonates may be an interesting new line.

Clinical studies

Despite a great number of studies showing the antiosteolytic effect and the wide clinical use of bisphosphonates in tumor-induced bone disease, it has for a long time been difficult to draw clear conclusions about which bisphosphonate to use in which patient as well as the optimal regimen to administer. This is due to many factors. First, as seen above, the disease is extremely heterogeneous with respect to the causative tumor and to the mechanisms involved. Therapy is also not necessarily identical for the various effects desired, such as the reduction of hypercalcemia, reduction of pain, or the prevention of new osteolytic foci. Furthermore many studies were not controlled, involved too few patients with too many different dosage regimens, or involved other treatments, especially chemotherapy, so that valid conclusions could often not be drawn. Lastly, many studies, especially the early ones, used rehydration together with the bisphosphonate, so that it was not always possible to draw reliable conclusions about the relative effect of the two.

Effects

The great majority of studies have been performed with clodronate and pamidronate, fewer with etidronate. As with Paget's disease, it seems that the main differences between the different compounds are their respective potencies.

Mechanisms of
hypercalcemia
pp. 87–89

Bisphosphonates are very effective in decreasing calcemia. With intravenous administration, the effect starts to be significant after 2–3 days, normocalcemia being obtained after 3–5 days and the full effect after about a week. As discussed above, the effect is most pronounced in patients in whom hypercalcemia is completely or largely a result of bone resorption only, as is the case, for example, in myeloma. Hypocalcemia can occur in some rare cases, but is usually without symptoms.

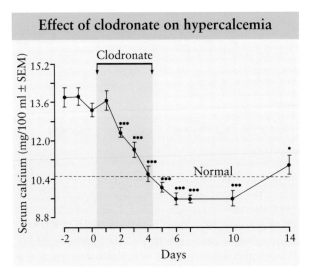

Fig. 3.3-8 Effect of clodronate infused in most cases for 5 days intravenously at a dose of 300 mg on hypercalcemia of malignancy. *$p < 0.01$; ***$p < 0.0001$. (Adapted from Urwin, G.H. *et al.* (1987). *Bone,* **8** (Suppl. 1), S43–S51, with kind permission from the author and Pergamon Press Ltd., Headington Hill Hall, Oxford, OX3, 0BW, UK.)

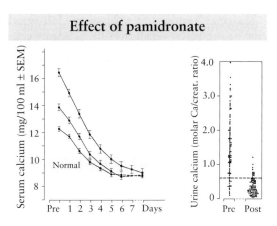

Fig. 3.3-9 Effect of pamidronate given daily at 15 mg intravenously for up to 10 days on calcemia and calciuria in hypercalcemia of malignancy. (Adapted from Harinck, H.I.J. *et al.* (1987). Reproduced from *Am. J. Med.*, **82**, 1133–42, with copyright permission from the author and the publisher.)

Bisphosphonates are also effective in carcinoma of the parathyroid, although their effect is only of short duration after discontinuation of treatment, as discussed in the next chapter.

Hyperparathyroidism p. 112

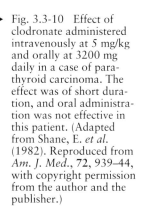

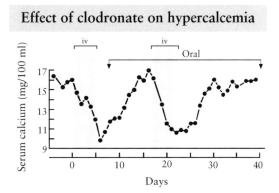

Fig. 3.3-10 Effect of clodronate administered intravenously at 5 mg/kg and orally at 3200 mg daily in a case of parathyroid carcinoma. The effect was of short duration, and oral administration was not effective in this patient. (Adapted from Shane, E. *et al.* (1982). Reproduced from *Am. J. Med.*, **72**, 939–44, with copyright permission from the author and the publisher.)

Bisphosphonates decrease and often normalize plasma calcium.

With clodronate and pamidronate, plasma phosphate and tubular reabsorption of phosphate can decrease, as seen in Paget's disease. This might be, at least partially, the consequence of the observed increase in previously suppressed parathyroid hormone. In contrast, plasma phosphate may increase with etidronate, as is also the case with this bisphosphonate in other indications. While parathyroid hormone and 1,25 $(OH)_2$ vitamin D are increased under treatment with bisphosphonate, the levels of PTH-related peptide are not altered.

Etidronate and plasma phosphate p. 149

Calciuria is greatly decreased in all types of tumor. Urinary hydroxy-proline is also diminished, although sometimes less than predicted. The reason for this is unclear and has been attributed to tumor-induced non-osseous collagen turnover in soft tissues, a process that is not influenced by bisphosphonates. This discrepancy should not be present when the urinary crosslinks from bone are measured (*see* Figs. 3.3-11–3.3-13).

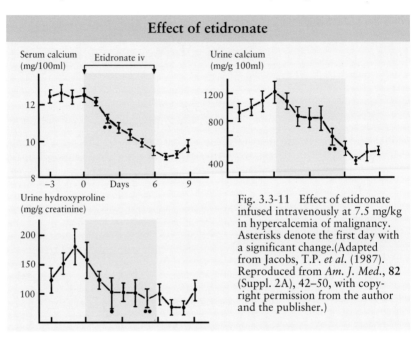

Effect of etidronate

Fig. 3.3-11   Effect of etidronate infused intravenously at 7.5 mg/kg in hypercalcemia of malignancy. Asterisks denote the first day with a significant change.(Adapted from Jacobs, T.P. *et al.* (1987). Reproduced from *Am. J. Med.*, **82** (Suppl. 2A), 42–50, with copyright permission from the author and the publisher.)

Serum alkaline phosphatase is usually unchanged, at least acutely, showing that the effect of the drug is on the resorption process. Finally, renal function can improve.

Urinary calcium is often normalized. Urinary hydroxyproline is diminished but less than expected, possibly because of soft tissue involvement, which is not influenced by bisphosphonates.

The duration of the effect after discontinuation of the drug is difficult to assess. The time to recurrence varies greatly from patient to patient, and depends upon the type of tumor, the dosage and the compound used. The effect lasts longer in focal bone disease, such as in the presence of metastases. This has been explained by the preferential deposition of bisphosphonates in the locations invaded by the tumor cells. In contrast, recurrence occurs much faster when bone resorption is more generalized,

Effect of clodronate

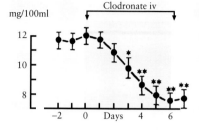

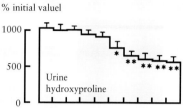

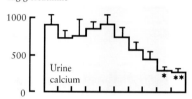

3.3-12 Effect of 5 mg/kg of clodronate given intravenously for 6 days in hypercalcemia of malignancy. (Adapted and reproduced with permission from Jacobs, T.P. *et al.* (1981). Hypercalcemia of malignancy: treatment with intravenous dichloromethylene diphosphonate. *Ann. Intern. Med.*, **94**, 312–16.)

Fig. 3.3-13 Effect of a median dose of 0.5 (0.25–0.75), 1.0 (exactly), and 1.5 (1.25–4.5) mg/kg of pamidronate administered intravenously for 1–3 days in 160 hypercalcemic tumor patients. (Adapted from Body, J.J. and Dumon, J.C. (1994). *Ann. Oncol.*, 5. 359–63. Reproduced with permission from the author and the publisher.)

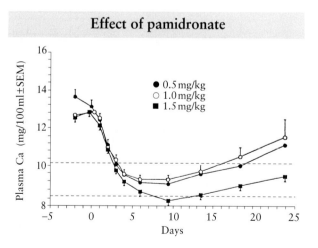

Effect of pamidronate

Parathyroid
carcinoma
pp. 112–113

such as in humoral hypercalcemia of malignancy or carcinoma of the parathyroid. In general recurrence is seen between a few days and 1 month, sometimes more. If therapy is resumed, the effect is usually obtained again. The most practical procedure is therefore to monitor calcemia and calciuria and to resume treatment when blood calcium increases again.

> *The duration of the effect after discontinuation of treatment is variable, usually less than a month. It seems to depend upon the potency of the bisphosphonate, the total dose administered and the type of bone disease. In patients with focal involvement, resorption appears to be inhibited for longer than in those with humoral hypercalcemia.*

Bisphosphonates, at least clodronate and pamidronate, diminish bone pain, leading sometimes to a marked improvement in the quality of life. Under chronic therapy they also decrease the occurrence of fractures and the appearance of new osteolytic foci in both myeloma and metastatic disease although, as expected, the development of metastases in soft tissues is not altered. The effects are lost after discontinuation of the drug. In view of these results, treatment to prevent skeletal metastases in primary tumors with a frequent skeletal dissemination, such as carcinoma of the breast, becomes an interesting possibility.

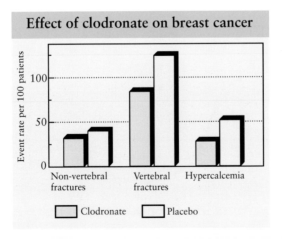

Fig. 3.3-14 Effect of 1600 mg of clodronate given daily for up to 18 months on skeletal complications in patients with carcinoma of the breast. (Adapted from Paterson, A.H.G. *et al.* (1993). Picture courtesy of Dr J.A. Kanis.)

Fig. 3.3-15 Effect of 300 mg of pamidronate given daily orally on the cumulative sum of complications in tumor bone disease. (Adapted from van Holten-Verzantvoort, A.T.M. *et al.* (1993). Reproduced with permission from the author and W.B. Saunders.)

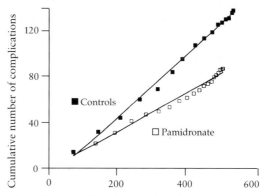

Effect of pamidronate on complications

Cumulative number of 3-month evaluation periods

Clodronate and pamidronate decrease bone pain, and diminish the development of new osteolytic foci and the occurrence of fractures.

Various bisphosphonates, such as clodronate, pamidronate and recently also risedronate are effective also in multiple myeloma. In this disease they decrease calcemia and the number of hypercalcemic episodes, bone resorption, bone pain, the number of fractures and the number of radiotherapy courses, and prevent skeletal deterioration.

Bisphosphonates are effective also in multiple myeloma.

Treatment regimens

One should distinguish between the treatment of hypercalcemia, treatment directed towards a long-term decrease of new osteolytic lesions and fractures, and an improvement in the quality of life.

Hypercalcemia is usually treated by intravenous administration of the bisphosphonate until blood calcium reaches a plateau. If this plateau is higher than desired, it is possible either to increase the dose, if this is acceptable from the toxicological point of view, or to change to a more powerful compound. Once the desired calcemia is reached, the administration is discontinued until serum calcium increases again to an unacceptable level.

Clodronate

For the treatment of patients with hypercalcemia, 300 mg of clodronate given as an intravenous infusion daily for about 5 days is very efficacious. It appears that the total dose is relevant, one infusion of 1500 mg being as effective as five infusions of 300 mg. Certain centers use 300 mg/day for 2–3 days or 600 mg for 1 day, which appears to be a good choice. An effect can also be seen by administering clodronate orally, but a high dose, generally 1600–3200 mg/day, is needed. However, since the decrease in calcemia is slower, this treatment cannot be given in emergency cases.

> *Intravenous infusions of 300 mg/day of clodronate for 5 days are usually given. A single infusion of 600 mg or more for 1 day is also effective.*

Paget's
disease
p. 78

The duration of the effect is very variable, relapse usually occurring within a month. As in Paget's disease, it appears that the duration is related not only to the severity of the disease, but also to the total administered dose.

Treatment should be resumed when calcemia rises again. Another possibility is to administer clodronate orally as maintenance therapy after the initial intravenous treatment. After a start with 800 mg daily, the dose can be increased to 1600 mg or even 3200 mg orally if the desired effect is not obtained. However, this treatment is not efficacious in all patients, even at the highest doses.

> *For long-term therapy of hypercalcemia, one can use either repeated courses of intravenous infusions, or oral administration of 800–3200 mg daily.*

Effect on
complications
pp. 98–99

For the long-term therapy of other complications of tumor bone disease, the daily oral administration of 1600 mg clodronate has been shown to reduce the formation of new osteolytic lesions, the further growth of existing lesions and the occurrence of fractures. The results of a first study have been recently confirmed in a larger multicenter trial. Similar effects have been obtained in myeloma using 2400 mg daily.

> *Chronic oral administration of 1600–2400 mg of clodronate daily is effective in the prevention of new osteolytic foci and fractures.*

All these doses have been developed with clodronate administered in the form of capsules. Very recently a new galenic presentation, namely film-coated tablets, which show an approximate 50% increase in biovailability, has been developed by one of the producers. With these tablets, a daily dose of 1040 mg is suggested.

> **When clodronate is administered as film coated tablets, a dose of 1040 mg daily is effective**

Etidronate

Although the first report of the effect of etidronate on tumor-induced bone disease was published in 1980 and the activity was then confirmed by later investigations, the number of studies are fewer than those with clodronate and pamidronate. Nearly all patients have received the same dose of 7.5 mg/kg intravenously, given mostly for 3 days, in fewer cases somewhat longer. The compound is diluted in about 500 ml of liquid and administered over a few hours, in order to prevent precipitation or the formation of aggregates.

Intravenous administration p. 146

This dose leads to a normalization of calcemia in 7–10 days in a quarter of the patients, longer treatments being apparently somewhat more effective. The effect disappears within a month, sometimes already within days after discontinuation of the drug. If the effect is not satisfactory, or if calcemia rises again, the treatment can be repeated after an interval of 1 week. However, the long-term effect of repeated dosing on bone mineralization is unknown. There are only few results with regimens other than this, so that it is not known whether improvement is possible. Among the various bisphosphonates used, the effect of etidronate, being the least potent, appears the least satisfactory.

> **Etidronate given at 7.5 mg/kg intravenously for 3 days can decrease hypercalcemia, as well as calciuria and hydroxyprolinuria. Its effect is weaker than that of the other bisphosphonates used.**

Pamidronate

Most studies have been performed using intravenous infusions, and many different doses for different durations have been tried. When it was realized that similar effects can be obtained when the same total dose is given once instead of divided over several days, the protocol with a single infusion gained popularity. The optimal dose ranges between 15 and 90 mg and should be adapted to the initial hypercalcemia, severely hypercalcemic patients requiring the larger dose. Thus, 15–30 mg is usually sufficient for calcemias up to 12 mg/100 ml, while 30–60 mg is suggested for calcemias between 12 and 14 mg/100 ml, 60–90 mg for calcemias between 14 and 16 mg/100 ml, and 90 mg for calcemias above 16 mg/100 ml. For the sake of simplicity many centers today use only 60 mg for calcemia levels below 13 mg/100 ml and 90 mg for calcemias above this concentration. When correctly dosed, normocalcemia can be obtained in 90% or more of the cases. As for the other bisphosphonates, treatment is resumed when blood calcium increases again. The compound must always be dissolved in 250 ml for up to 60 mg and in 500 ml for up to 90 mg and be infused not faster than in 1 h and 2 h, respectively. In myeloma an infusion time of 4 h is recommended.

> *One infusion of pamidronate is usually sufficient to normalize calcemia in hypercalcemia. The dose should be adapted to the degree of hypercalcemia and lies between 30 and 90 mg. Treatment is repeated when calcemia rises again.*

Various trials have adressed the question of the optimal chronic therapy to prevent the development of fractures and of new osteolytic foci and other complications. Doses between 45 and 90 mg every 3–4 weeks, given in a single infusion, were shown to slow down the progression of the skeletal disease and to reduce bone pain. In patients with advanced disease, 60–90 mg is suggested. Doses of 20 mg/week were necessary to improve pain. Chronic oral therapy with 300 mg daily has also been found to be effective, but is often accompanied by gastrointestinal side effects. To our knowledge, oral pamidronate is not commercially available at the present time, with the exception of a few countries in South America.

Adverse events p. 151

Commercially available bisphosphonates pp. 157–170

> *For chronic therapy to prevent complications, infusions of 45–90 mg every 3–4 weeks are suggested. Oral treatment with 300 mg daily is effective, but can be accompanied by gastrointestinal side events. Furthermore, oral formulations are practically unavailable commercially.*

Other bisphosphonates

Chemical structures pp. 35–36

Data on other bisphosphonates are still scanty. When investigated for the calcium-lowering effect, tiludronate has an activity similar to that of etidronate. Neridronate was found to be effective with one infusion of 125 mg. Cimadronate was effective at 10 mg, alendronate being very active at this dosage. The same was true for ibandronate, which is active at a single dose of 2–6 mg. Risedronate decreased bone resorption in myeloma when given orally at 30 mg daily for 6 months.

Fig. 3.3-16 Effect of a single infusion of alendronate in tumor hypercalcemia. Some patients given the lower doses received a second infusion on day 3. (Adapted from Rizzoli, R. *et al.* (1992). *Int. J. Cancer*, 50, 706–12. Reproduced with permission from the author and publisher.)

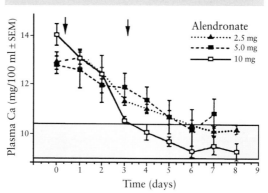

Alendronate, cimadronate and ibandronate are on a milligram basis the most potent bisphosphonates in hypercalcemia of malignancy.

Comparison of the various bisphosphonates

From the available data, there is no indication that there are any fundamental differences in the qualitative effect of the various bisphosphonates in tumor-induced bone disease. There is, however, a great difference in the quantitative effect. From the results reported above, it appears that the total parenteral dose of bisphosphonate effective in reducing calcemia in tumor-induced bone disease ranges from roughly 1 to over 1000. It is of interest that the sequence as well as the range of potency, as defined by the amount of drug necessary to reduce calcemia found in humans, are not far from those observed in the rat.

Potency in rat p. 44

Fig. 3.3-17 Approximate relative activity of various bisphosphonates in tumoral hypercalcemia.

Relative activity in humans

Etidronate   1
Clodronate
Neridronate
Pamidronate
Climadronate
Alendronate
Ibandronte   >1000

The activity increases from 1 to 1000 in the sequence etidronate, clodronate, neridronate, pamidronate, cimadronate, alendronate, ibandronate.

Since a more potent substance is not necessarily a better one, it is difficult to decide which bisphosphonate to use if more than one is available. From the three commercially available, etidronate, clodronate and pamidronate, the first appears to be the least suitable. Because of its relatively low activity, it is not always efficacious. Furthermore the effective doses are those that can lead to an inhibition of normal mineralization, a potential drawback if therapy is of long duration. Therefore, if available, the other two should be preferred. Between clodronate and pamidronate, both are good choices, the latter appearing to have a somewhat more sustained effect, at least at the doses investigated up to now. However, clodronate is better tolerated when given orally, at least with the formulations of pamidronate used in the past. Furthermore, to our knowledge, no commercial oral pamidronate preparation is yet available in most countries. Thus, clodronate is the choice when oral administration is desired.

Commercially available bisphosphonates pp. 157–170

Clodronate and pamidronate appear to be the compounds of choice today. In the acute treatment of hypercalcemia both are active, pamidronate being apparently somewhat longer acting. For chronic treatment of hypercalcemia and of the other complications, clodronate is preferred if oral therapy is desired. If neither of these is available, intravenous etidronate can also be useful.

Conclusion

Today bisphosphonates are the drugs of choice to treat tumor bone disease. By inhibiting bone resorption, they correct hypercalcemia, reduce pain, prevent the development of new osteolytic lesions, the occurrence of fractures and in consequence improve the quality of life. Clodronate and pamidronate, and to a certain extent etidronate, are commercially available for this indication in many countries.

Recommended selected reading

Tumor bone disease

Reviews

Bilezikian, J.P. (1992). Drug therapy: management of acute hypercalcemia. *N. Engl. J. Med.*, **326**, 1196–203

Kanis, J.A., Cundy, T., Heynen, G. and Russell, R.G.G. (1980). The pathophysiology of hypercalcemia. *Metab. Bone Dis. Relat. Res.*, **2**, 151–9

Martin, T.J., Moseley, J.M. and Gillespie, M.T. (1991). Parathyroid hormone-related protein: biochemistry and molecular biology. *Crit. Rev. Biochem. Mol. Biol.*, **26**, 377–95

Mosekilde, L., Eriksen, E.F. and Charles, P. (1991). Hypercalcemia of malignancy: pathophysiology, diagnosis and treatment. *Crit. Rev. Oncol. Hematol.*, **11**, 1–27

Mundy, G.R. and Martin, T.J. (1993). Pathophysiology of skeletal complications of cancer. In Mundy, G.R. and Martin, T.J. (eds.) *Physiology and Pharmacology of Bone. Handbook of Experimental Pharmacology*, vol. 107, pp. 641–71

Orloff, J.J. and Stewart, A.F. (1992). Disorders of serum minerals caused by cancer. In Coe, F.L. and Favus, M.J. (eds.) *Disorders of Bone and Mineral Metabolism*, pp. 539–62. (New York: Raven Press)

Ralston, S.H. (1990). The pathogenesis of humoral hypercalcemia of malignancy. In Heersche, J.N.M. and Kanis, J.A. (eds.) *Bone and Mineral Research*, vol. 7, pp. 139–73. (Amsterdam, New York, Oxford: Elsevier)

Stewart, A.F. and Broadus, A.E. (1990). Clinical review 16: parathyroid hormone-related proteins: coming of age in the 1990s. *J. Clin. Endocrinol. Metab.*, **71**, 1410–14

Wimalawansa, S.J. (ed) (1995). *Hypercalcemia of Malignancy, Etiology, Pathogenesis and Clinical Management.* (Berlin, Germany, and Austin, USA: Springer)

Bisphosphonates, preclinical

Review

Fleisch, H. (1991). Bisphosphonates. Pharmacology and use in the treatment of tumour-induced hypercalcaemic and metastatic bone disease. *Drugs*, **42**, 919–44

Original articles

Guaitani, A., Polentarutti, N., Filippeschi, S., Marmonti, L., Corti, F., Italia, C., Coccioli, G., Donelli, M.G., Mantovani, A. and Garattini, S. (1984). Effects of disodium etidronate in murine tumor models. *Eur. J. Cancer Clin. Oncol.*, **20**, 685–93

Hall, D.G. and Stoica, G. (1994). Effect of the bisphosphonate risedronate on bone metastases in a rat mammary adenocarcinoma model system. *J. Bone Miner. Res.*, **9**, 221–30

Jung, A., Bornand, J., Mermillod, B., Edouard, C. and Meunier, P.J. (1984). Inhibition by diphosphonates of bone resorption induced by the Walker tumor of the rat. *Cancer Res.*, **44**, 3007–11

Jung, A., Mermillod, B., Barras, C., Baud, M. and Courvoisier, B. (1981). Inhibition by two diphosphonates of bone lysis in tumor-conditioned media. *Cancer Res.*, **41**, 3233–7

Martodam, R.R., Thornton, K.S., Sica, D.A., D'Souza, S.M., Flora, L. and Mundy, G.R. (1983). The effects of dichloromethylene diphosphonate on hypercalcemia and other parameters of the humoral hypercalcemia of malignancy in the rat Leydig cell tumor. *Calcif. Tissue Int.*, **35**, 512–19

Sturtz, G., Couthon, H., Fabulet, O., Mian, M. and Rosini, S. (1993). Synthesis of gem-bis-phosphonic methotrexate conjugates and their biological response towards Walker's osteosarcoma. *Eur. J. Med. Chem.*, **28**, 899–903

Bisphosphonates, clinical

Review

Fleisch, H. (1991). Bisphosphonates. Pharmacology and use in the treatment of tumour-induced hypercalcaemic and metastatic bone disease. *Drugs*, **42**, 919–44

Alendronate

Original articles

Adami, S., Bolzicco, G.P., Rizzo, A., Salvagno, G., Bertoldo, F., Rosini, M., Suppi, R. and Lo Cascio, V. (1987). The use of dichloromethylene bisphosphonate and aminobutane bisphosphonate in hypercalcemia of malignancy. *Bone Miner.*, **2**, 395–404

Nussbaum, S.R., Warrell, R.P. Jr, Rude, R., Glusman, J., Bilezikian, J.P., Stewart, A.F., Stepanavage, M., Sacco, J.F., Averbuch, S.D. and Gertz, B.J. (1993). Dose–response study of alendronate sodium for the treatment of cancer-associated hypercalcemia. *J. Clin. Oncol.*, **11**, 1618–23

Rizzoli, R., Buchs, B. and Bonjour, J.-P. (1992). Effect of a single infusion of alendronate in malignant hypercalcaemia: dose dependency and comparison with clodronate. *Int. J. Cancer*, **50**, 706–12

Clodronate

Reviews

Hannuniemi, R., Laurén, L. and Puolijoki, H. (1991). Clodronate: an effective agent for the treatment of increased bone resorption. *Drugs Today*, **27**, 375–90

Kanis, J.A., O'Rourke, N. and McCloskey, E.V. (1994). Consequences of neoplasia induced bone resorption and the use of clodronate. *Int. J. Oncol.*, **5**, 713–31

Müsel, B. and Scigalla, P. (1992). Pharmacology and clinical use of bisphosphonates in oncology. *Onkologie*, **15**, 444–53

Plosker, G.L. and Goa, K.L. (1994). Clodronate. A review of its pharmacological proper-ties and therapeutic efficacy in resorptive bone disease. *Drugs*, **47**, 945–82

Original articles

Delmas, P.D., Charhon, S., Chapuy, M.C., Vignon, E., Briançon, D., Edouard, C. and Meunier, P.J. (1982). Long-term effects of dichloromethylene diphosphonate (Cl_2MDP) on skeletal lesions in multiple myeloma. *Metab. Bone Dis. Relat. Res.*, **4**, 163–8

Douglas, D.L., Duckworth, T., Russell, R.G.G., Kanis, J.A., Preston, C.J., Preston, F.E., Prenton, M.A. and Woodhead, J.S. (1980). Effect of dichloromethylene diphosphonate in Paget's disease of bone and in hypercalcaemia due to primary hyperparathyroidism or malignant disease. *Lancet*, **1**, 1043–7

Elomaa, I., Blomqvist, C., Gröhn, P., Porkka, L., Kairento, A.L., Selander, K., Lamberg-Allardt, C. and Holmström, T. (1983). Long-term controlled trial with diphosphonate in patients with osteolytic bone metastases. *Lancet*, **1**, 146–9

Jacobs, T.P., Siris, E.S., Bilezikian, J.P., Baquiran, D.C., Shane, E. and Canfield, R.E. (1981). Hypercalcemia of malignancy: treatment with intravenous dichloromethylene diphosphonate. *Ann. Intern. Med.*, **94**, 312–16

Lahtinen, R., Laakso, M., Palva, I., Virkkunen, P. and Elomaa, I. (1992). Randomised, placebo-controlled multicentre trial of clodronate in multiple myeloma. *Lancet*, **340**, 1049–52

O'Rourke, N.P., McCloskey, E.V., Vasikaran, S., Eyres, K., Fern, D. and Kanis, J.A. (1993). Effective treatment of malignant hypercalcaemia with a single intravenous infusion of clodronate. *Br. J. Cancer*, **67**, 560–3

Paterson, A.H.G., Powles, T.J., Kanis, J.A., McCloskey, E., Hanson, J. and Ashley, S. (1993). Double-blind controlled trial of oral clodronate in patients with bone metastases from breast cancer. *J. Clin. Oncol.*, **11**, 59–65

Shane, E., Jacobs, T.P., Siris, E.S., Steinberg, S.F., Stoddart, K., Canfield, R.E. and Bilezikian, J.P. (1982). Therapy of hypercalcemia due to parathyroid carcinoma with intravenous dichloromethylene diphosphonate. *Am. J. Med.*, **72**, 939–44

Siris, E.S., Sherman, W.H., Baquiran, D.C., Schlatterer, J.P., Osserman, E.F. and Canfield, R.E. (1980). Effects of dichloromethylene diphosphonate on skeletal mobilization of calcium in multiple myeloma. *N. Engl. J. Med.*, **302**, 310–15

Urwin, G.H., Yates, A.J.P., Gray, R.E.S., Hamdy, N.A.T., McCloskey, E.V., Preston, F.E., Greaves, M., Neil, F.E. and Kanis, J.A. (1987). Treatment of the hypercalcaemia of malignancy with intravenous clodronate. *Bone*, **8** (Suppl 1), S43–S51

Etidronate

Symposium

(1987). Etidronate disodium: a new therapy for hypercalcemia of malignancy. Proceedings of a symposium. *Am. J. Med.*, **82** (Suppl. 2A), 1–78

Review

Dunn, C.J., Fitton, A. and Sorkin, E.M. (1994). Etidronic acid. A review of its pharmacological properties and therapeutic efficacy in resorptive bone disease. *Drugs Aging*, **5**, 446–74

Original articles

Gucalp, R., Ritch, P., Wiernik, P.H., Sarma, P.R., Keller, A., Richman, S.P., Tauer, K., Neidhart, J., Mallette, L.E., Siegel, R. and VandePol, C.J. (1992). Comparative study of pamidronate and etidronate disodium in the treatment of cancer-related hypercalcemia. *J. Clin. Oncol.*, **10**, 134–42

Jacobs, T.P., Gordon, A.C., Silverberg, S.J., Shane, E., Reich, L., Clemens, T.L. and Gundberg, C.H. (1987). Neoplastic hypercalcemia: physiologic response to intravenous etidronate disodium. *Am. J. Med.*, **82** (Suppl. 2A), 42–50

Jung, A. (1982). Comparison of two parenteral diphosphonates in hypercalcemia of malignancy. *Am. J. Med.*, **72**, 221–6

Kanis, J.A., Urwin, G.H., Gray, R.E.S., Beneton, M.N.C., McCloskey, E.V., Hamdy, N.A.T. and Murray, S.A. (1987). Effects of intravenous etidronate disodium on skeletal and calcium metabolism. *Am. J. Med.*, **82** (Suppl. 2A), 55–70

Ryzen, E., Martodam, R.R., Troxell, M., Benson, A., Paterson, A., Shepard, K. and Hicks, R. (1985). Intravenous etidronate in the management of malignant hypercalcemia. *Arch. Intern. Med.*, **145**, 449–52

Singer, F.R., Ritch, P.S., Lad, T.E., Ringenberg, Q.S., Schiller, J.H., Recker, R.R. and Ryzen, E. (1991). Treatment of hypercalcemia of malignancy with intravenous etidronate. A controlled, multicenter study. *Arch. Intern. Med.*, **151**, 471–6

Pamidronate

Symposia

Burckhardt, P. (ed.) (1989). *Disodium Pamidronate (APD) in the Treatment of Malignancy-Related Disorders.* (Toronto, Lewiston NY, Bern, Stuttgart: Hans Huber Publishers)
Goldhirsch, A. (ed.) (1994). Progress in the treatment and palliation of advanced breast cancer. *Ann. Oncol.*, **5** (Suppl.7, Part 2), 25–55

Reviews

Fitton, A. and McTavish, D. (1991). Pamidronate: a review of its pharmacological properties and therapeutic efficacy in resorptive bone disease. *Drugs*, **41**, 289–318
Kellihan, M.J. and Mangino, P.D. (1992). Pamidronate. *Ann. Pharmocotherapy*, **26**, 1262–9

Original articles

Body, J.J. and Dumon, J.C. (1994). Treatment of tumour-induced hypercalcaemia with the bisphosphonate pamidronate: dose–response relationship and influence of tumour type. *Ann. Oncol.*, **5**, 359–63
Body, J.-J., Magritte, A., Seraj, F., Sculier, J.P. and Borkowski, A. (1989). Aminohydroxypropylidene bisphosphonate (APD) treatment for tumor-associated hypercalcemia: a randomized comparison between a 3-day treatment and single 24-hour infusions. *J. Bone Miner. Res.*, **4**, 923–8
Body, J.-J., Pot, M., Borkowski, A., Sculier, J.P. and Klastersky, J. (1987). Dose/response study of aminohydroxypropylidene bisphosphonate in tumor associated hypercalcemia. *Am. J. Med.*, **82**, 957–63
Conte, P.F., Giannessi, P.G., Latreille, J., Mauriac, L., Koliren, L., Calabresi, F. and Ford, J.M. (1994). Delayed progression of bone metastases with pamidronate therapy in breast cancer patients: a randomized, multicenter phase III trial. *Ann. Oncol.*, **5** (Suppl. 7), S41–4
Glover, D., Lipton, A., Keller, A., Miller, A.A., Browning, S., Fram, R.J., George, S., Zelenakas, K., Macerata, R.S. and Seaman, J.J. (1994). Intravenous pamidronate disodium treatment of bone metastases in patients with breast cancer. *Cancer*, **74**, 2949–55
Gucalp, R., Ritch, P., Wiernik, P.H., Sarma, P.R., Keller, A., Richman, S.P., Tauer, K., Neidhart, J., Mallette, L.E., Siegel, R. and VandePol, C.J. (1992). Comparative study of pamidronate and etidronate disodium in the treatment of cancer-related hypercalcemia. *J. Clin. Oncol.*, **10**, 134–42
Harinck, H.I.J., Bijvoet, O.L.M., Plantingh, A.S.T., Body, J.J., Elte, J.W.F., Sleeboom, H.P., Wildiers, J. and Neijt, J.P. (1987). Role of bone and kidney in tumor-induced hypercalcemia and its treatment with bisphosphonate and sodium chloride. *Am. J. Med.*, **82**, 1133–42
Nussbaum, S.R., Younger, J., VandePol, C.J., Gagel, R.F., Zubler, M.A., Chapman, R., Henderson, I.C. and Mallette, L.E. (1993). Single-dose intravenous therapy with pamidronate for the treatment of hypercalcemia of malignancy: comparison of 30-, 60-, and 90-mg dosages. *Am. J. Med.*, **95**, 297–304

Thiébaud, D., Jaeger, P., Jacquet, A.F. and Burckhardt, P. (1988). Dose–response in the treatment of hypercalcemia of malignancy by a single infusion of the bisphosphonate AHPrBP. *J. Clin. Oncol.*, **6**, 762–8

Thiébaud, D., Leyvraz, S., von Fliedner, V., Perey, L., Cornu, P., Thiébaud, S. and Burckhardt, P. (1991). Treatment of bone metastases from breast cancer and myeloma with pamidronate. *Eur. J. Cancer*, **27**, 37–41

Thiébaud, D., Portmann, L., Jaeger, P., Jacquet, A.F. and Burckhardt, P. (1986). Oral versus intravenous AHPrBP (APD) in the treatment of hypercalcemia of malignancy. *Bone*, **7**, 247–53

Thürlimann, B., Morant, R., Jungi, W.F. and Radziwill, A. (1994). Pamidronate for pain control in patients with malignant osteolytic bone disease: a prospective dose–effect study. *Support Care Cancer*, **2**, 61–5

van Breukelen, F.J.M., Bijvoet, O.L.M. and van Oosterom, A.T. (1979). Inhibition of osteolytic bone lesions by (3-amino-1-hydroxypropylidene)-1,1-bisphosphonate (A.P.D.). *Lancet*, **1**, 803–5

van Holten-Verzantvoort, A.T.M., Kroon, H.M., Bijvoet, O.L.M., Cleton, F.J., Beex, L.V.A.M., Blijham, G., Hermans, J., Neijt, J.P., Papapoulos, S.E., Sleeboom, H.P., Vermey, P. and Zwinderman, A.H. (1993). Palliative pamidronate treatment in patients with bone metastases from breast cancer. *J. Clin. Oncol.*, **11**, 491–8

Tiludronate

Dumon, J.C., Magritte, A. and Body, J.J. (1991). Efficacy and safety of the bisphosphonate tiludronate for the treatment of tumor-associated hypercalcemia. *Bone Miner.*, **15**, 257–66

Other bisphosphonates

Fukumoto, S., Matsumoto, T., Takebe, K., Onaya, T., Eto, S., Nawata, H. and Ogata, E. (1994). Treatment of malignancy-associated hypercalcemia with YM175, a new bisphosphonate: elevated threshold for parathyroid hormone secretion in hypercalcemic patients. *J. Clin. Endocrinol. Metab.*, **79**, 165–70

O'Rourke, N.P., McCloskey, E.V., Rosini, S., Coleman, R.E. and Kanis, J.A. (1994). Treatment of malignant hypercalcemia with aminohexane bisphosphonate (neridronate). *Br. J. Cancer*, **69**, 914–17

Roux, C., Ravaud, P., Cohen-Solal, M., de Vernejoul, M.C., Guillemant, S., Cherruau, B., Delmas, P., Dougados, M. and Amor, B. (1994). Biologic, histologic and densitometric effects of oral risedronate on bone in patients with multiple myeloma. *Bone*, **15**, 41–9

Wüster, C., Schöter, K.H., Thiébaud, D., Manegold, C., Krahl, D., Clemens, M.R., Ghielmini, M., Jaeger, P. and Scharla, S.H. (1993). Methylpentylaminopropylidenebisphosphonate (BM 21.0955): a new potent and safe bisphosphonate for the treatment of cancer-associated hypercalcemia. *Bone Miner.*, **22**, 77–85

3.4. Non-tumor-induced hypercalcemia

3.4.1. Definition

All hypercalcemias due to causes other than malignant bone disease fall under this category.

3.4.2. Pathophysiology

Calcium homeostasis pp. 23–26 pp. 87–89

An increase in blood calcium can be due to an elevated flux of calcium from bone or the intestine, or due to an increase in the tubular reabsorption of calcium.

An increase in the calcium flux from bone, following elevated bone destruction, is by far the most common mechanism. Examples are hyperparathyroidism, the most frequent cause, thyrotoxicosis, granulomatous diseases such as sarcoidosis, vitamin D intoxication and certain cases of acute osteoporosis, as during immobilization. Increased intestinal calcium absorption is less frequent and contributes less to hypercalcemia. It occurs, for example, in vitamin D intoxication or in granulomatous disease with increased production of $1,25(OH)_2$ vitamin D.

PTH-related peptide p. 87

An increase in tubular reabsorption of calcium is usually due to abnormally high levels of parathyroid hormone or of PTH-related peptide. It is encountered in primary hyperparathyroidism or, as discussed in the preceding chapter, in certain tumors.

Often more than one mechanism is involved, such as in hyperparathyroidism, where the increase in blood calcium originates from both bone and kidney.

> *Hypercalcemia can result either from an increase in the flow of calcium from bone or the intestine to the blood, or from an increase in tubular reabsorption of calcium in the kidney.*

3.4.3. Clinical manifestations

Hypercalcemic syndrome p. 90

The clinical picture is that of the hypercalcemic syndrome. Disturbances involve the central and peripheral nervous system, the digestive and cardiovascular systems, the kidney and the muscles. Dangerous complications are the acute hypercalcemic crisis, which can be fatal, and ectopic calcification, which occurs especially in the kidney, where it can lead to renal failure, and in urine, leading to urolithiasis.

> *Hypercalcemia induces a large variety of disturbances and can be life threatening.*

3.4.4. Treatment with drugs other than bisphosphonates

Most hypercalcemias are relatively resistant to treatment other than that which is directed to the underlying disease. Drugs used include corticosteroids, prostaglandin inhibitors, calcitonin and furosemide, but the results are most often disappointing.

3.4.5. Treatment with bisphosphonates

Preclinical studies

The animal experiments which give the basis for the use of bisphosphonates in hypercalcemia in humans have been discussed extensively in the preclinical section. These compounds prevent or cure hypercalcemia induced by agents such as parathyroid hormone, vitamin D and its metabolites, and retinoids.

Bone
resorption
pp. 43–45

Fig 3.4-1 Effect of 10 mg P/kg of clodronate on the hypercalcemia induced in the rat by parathyroid extract. (Adapted from Fleisch, H., Russell, R.G.G. and Francis, M.D. (1969). Diphosphonates inhibit hydroxyapatite dissolution *in vitro* and bone resorption in tissue culture and *in vivo*. *Science*, **165**, 1262–4, with copyright permission from the author and the American Association for the Advancement of Science.)

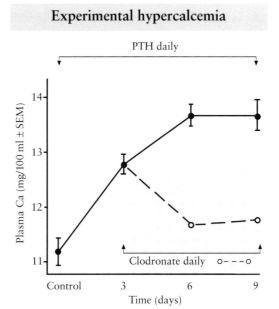

Bisphosphonates prevent or reverse hypercalcemia induced by various means in the animal.

Clinical studies

Only few data are available concerning the use of bisphosphonates in non-tumor-induced hypercalcemia. Most concern hyperparathyroidism.

Effects

Various bisphosphonates are active in decreasing serum calcium to some degree in some patients with hyperparathyroidism, both primary, secondary and tertiary. Some positive effects have also been seen in the hypercalcemia accompanying immobilization, thyrotoxicosis, sarcoidosis and vitamin D intoxication.

In general it appears that the bisphosphonates have only limited effects in the great majority of patients with non-tumor-induced hypercalcemia, especially those with hyperparathyroidism. This is not surprising, since the increase in serum calcium is due in most patients to an increase in parathyroid hormone, which acts to a large extent through the kidney.

Effect of PTH
p. 24

Furthermore, the bisphosphonates are not as long acting as, for example, in Paget's disease. It has been suggested that the long-lasting effect in this disease, as well as in other conditions with a focal involvement, is due to the specific accumulation of bisphosphonates at sites of focal resorption. They would be less active in diseases with generalized resorption, such as hyperparathyroidism, where new BMUs form constantly throughout the skeleton, so that the bisphosphonate will be present in a much lower concentration. Furthermore, new BMUs formed after cessation of treatment will not be exposed to the drug at all. It appears also that patients treated with more powerful bisphosphonates do normalize their fasting calcemia, but may become sensitive to calcium ingestion.

BMU
p. 22

> *Bisphosphonates are relatively less active on the hypercalcemia of hyperparathyroidism, because part of the elevation in serum calcium is due to the kidney. They are also active for a shorter time. Little is known about other diseases.*

Treatment regimens

Clodronate decreases calcemia when given intravenously at 300–600 mg daily or orally at 1600–3200 mg daily. Etidronate can be effective when given intravenously at 7.5 mg/kg daily, but appears mostly inactive when given orally. Also, pamidronate at 30 mg intravenously given as a single infusion, has shown activity. Daily oral doses of 20–40 mg of risedronate for 1 week are also effective. However, the effect of all compounds disappears relatively rapidly after discontinuation of treatment, so that it should be given continuously.

Parathyroid carcinoma
p. 95
p. 98

Clodronate, etidronate, pamidronate and risedronate can decrease calcemia in some cases of non-tumor-induced hypercalcemia. In general, dosages similar to those acting in tumor bone disease are recommended. In hyperparathyroidism the effect often disappears rapidly after discontinuation of treatment.

Conclusion

Bisphosphonates can occasionally be useful in non-tumor-induced hypercalcemia, but their effect, at least in hyperparathyroidism, is less than in tumor bone disease. Data in other diseases are scanty.

Recommended selected reading

Hypercalcemia

Reviews

Bilezikian, J.P. (1992). Hypercalcemic states: their differential diagnosis and acute management. In Coe, F.L. and Favus, M.J. (eds.) *Disorders of Bone and Mineral Metabolism*, pp. 493–521. (New York: Raven Press)

Breslau, N.A. and Pak, C.Y.C. (1992). Asymptomatic primary hyperparathyroidism. In Coe, F.L. and Favus, M.J. (eds.) *Disorders of Bone and Mineral Metabolism*, pp. 523–38. (New York: Raven Press)

Mundy, G.R. (1990). Primary hyperparathyroidism. Other causes of hypercalcemia. In Mundy, G.R. (ed.) *Calcium Homeostasis: Hypercalcemia and Hypocalcemia*, 2nd edn, pp. 137–95. (London: Martin Dunitz)

Peacock, M. (1993). Hyperparathyroid and hypoparathyroid bone disease. In Mundy, G.R. and Martin, T.J. (eds.) *Physiology and Pharmacology of Bone. Handbook of Experimental Pharmacology*, vol. 107, pp. 443–83. (Berlin, Heidelberg, New York: Springer-Verlag)

Reasner, C.A., Stone, M.D., Hosking, D.J., Ballah, A. and Mundy, G.R. (1993). Acute changes in calcium homeostasis during treatment of primary hyperparathyroidism with risedronate. *J. Clin. Endocrinol. Metab.*, 77, 1067–71

Original articles

Bisphosphonates, preclinical

Fleisch, H., Russell, R.G.G. and Francis, M.D. (1969). Diphosphonates inhibit hydroxy-apatite dissolution *in vitro* and bone resorption in tissue culture and *in vivo*. *Science*, **165**, 1262–4

Bisphosphonates, clinical

Hamdy, N.A.T., Gray, R.E.S., McCloskey, E., Galloway, J., Rattenbury, J.M., Brown, C.B. and Kanis, J.A. (1987). Clodronate in the medical management of hyperparathyroidism. *Bone*, **8** (Suppl. 1), S69–S77

Hamdy, N.A.T., McCloskey, E.V., Brown, C.B. and Kanis, J.A. (1990). Effects of clodronate in severe hyperparathyroid bone disease in chronic renal failure. *Nephron*, **56**, 6–12

Reasner, C.A., Stone, M.D., Hosking, D.J., Ballah, A. and Mundy, G.R. (1993). Acute changes in calcium homeostasis during treatment of primary hyperparathyroidism with risedronate. *J. Clin. Endocrinol. Metab.*, **77**, 1067–71

Rizzoli, R., Stoermann, C., Ammann, P. and Bonjour, J.-P. (1994). Hypercalcemia and hyperosteolysis in vitamin D intoxication: effects of clodronate therapy. *Bone*, **15**, 193–8

Shane, E., Baquiran, D.C. and Bilezikian, J.P. (1981). Effect of dichloromethylene diphosphonate on serum and urinary calcium in primary hyperparathyroidism. *Ann. Intern. Med.*, **95**, 23–7

3.5. Osteoporosis

3.5.1. Definition

Osteoporosis is a disease characterized by a decrease in bone mass and a deterioration in bone microarchitecture, which leads to an enhanced fragility of the skeleton and, therefore, to a greater risk of fracture. Recently a study group of the WHO has quantified this definition. Osteoporosis is present when the bone mineral density or bone mineral content is over 2.5 standard deviations below the young adult reference mean in the same sex (−2.5 T-scores). Furthermore, if fractures are present, the condition is called 'severe osteoporosis'.

Fig. 3.5-1 Definition of osteoporosis.

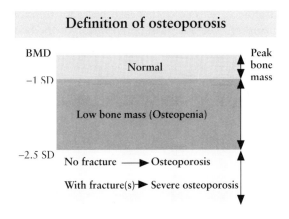

Per definition osteoporosis is present when the bone mass is over 2.5 standard deviations below that of the young adult.

3.5.2. Epidemiology

Osteoporosis is a very common disorder which will become even more common with the increase of life expectancy. The incidence is much higher in women than in men, and higher in whites and Asians than in blacks. It is estimated that up to four women out of ten who have reached the age of 50 will sustain in their life an osteoporotic fracture. This disease is, and will become even more so, a major public health issue, because of its medical and socioeconomic impact on our society. Development of preventive and curative treatment will thus be a main concern in the future.

Osteoporosis is a very common condition, especially in women.

3.5.3. Pathophysiology

During their lifetime, men lose on the average 20–30% of their maximum (peak) bone mass, women about 30–40%. The decrease in bone mass affects both cancellous and cortical bone, the former being more involved. It has been estimated that women lose about 50% of their cancellous bone and 30% of their cortical bone.

The trabeculae become thinner in women after menopause, also discontinuous and eventually even disappear, thus leading to a change in architecture. The cortex also becomes thinner and can show increased porosity. The chemical composition of the bone is not altered, however, in contrast to osteomalacia, which is primarily a defect of mineralization. In older people, both osteoporosis and osteomalacia may be present together, which explains, at least inpart why certain patients often respond astonishingly well to vitamin D and its derivatives

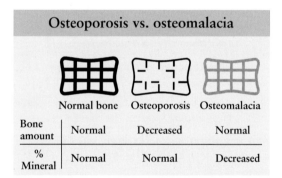

Osteoporosis vs. osteomalacia

	Normal bone	Osteoporosis	Osteomalacia
Bone amount	Normal	Decreased	Normal
% Mineral	Normal	Normal	Decreased

Fig. 3.5-2 The difference between osteoporosis and osteomalacia.

Osteoporosis is characterized by a loss of cancellous and cortical bone.

The loss of bone has a dual pattern. One is a continuous linear decrease in bone mass occurring in both women and men of about 0.5–1% a year, continuing until death. The age at which this loss starts is still disputed. While it is generally recognized that it is around age 50, some believe that it occurs earlier, at least in cancellous bone. In women, there is an additional rapid bone loss of variable intensity, up to a few per cent a year, and of variable length after the menopause, due to the decrease in estrogen production. After a certain time, bone mass will have reached a value where the structure becomes fragile and fractures occur. Since this takes place sooner in women than in men, they will also develop fractures earlier in life.

Fig. 3.5-3 Evolution of bone mass with age.

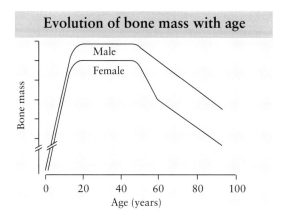

Evolution of bone mass with age

Male

Female

Bone mass

0   20   40   60   80   100

Age (years)

The main cause of osteoporosis is the continuous loss of bone during life, which is exacerbated in women after the menopause.

The second reason for osteoporosis, present in some patients, is a lesser bone production during adolescence. The maximum bone mass reached in life, called the peak bone mass, is attained at the end of the second decade. Women form a total bone mass which is inferior to that of men, since the outer volume of the bones is smaller. However, the true bone density is not smaller than that of men. The relative role of the two parameters, total bone mass and bone density for mechanical strength is not yet clear. The peak bone mass is determined mainly by heredity, possibly in part through the vitamin D receptor gene, and to a smaller extent by other factors such as nutrition. Calcium intake during youth may play a role, giving the rationale for the administration of calcium during growth. Since people with a smaller peak bone mass have less bone to start with, they will reach the fracture threshold earlier in the course of later bone loss.

The second contributory factor to the development of osteoporosis is the formation of too small a bone mass during adolescence.

Fig. 3.5-4 Mechanisms leading to osteoporosis.

Causes of osteoporosis

- Increase bone loss
- Too little peak bone mass

> *Osteoporosis can be due to increased bone loss, too little bone built during adolescence, or both. Women are more prone to osteoporosis, because of the rapid loss after the menopause.*

A distinction used to be made, although this is somewhat artificial, between postmenopausal osteoporosis and senile osteoporosis. The former is seen, as its name implies, after the menopause and has a greater effect on cancellous bone. In contrast the latter, encountered after the age of 70, involves both cancellous and cortical bone. Sometimes osteoporosis is the consequence of other diseases, such as hypercorticosteroidism ← or medical administration of corticosteroids, hyperthyroidism, hypogonadism, liver diseases, malignant diseases and immobilization. It is then called secondary osteoporosis.

> *One can distinguish between postmenopausal and senile osteoporosis, and osteoporosis secondary to other diseases.*

Bone resorption
p. 19

Calcium
homeostasis
p. 25
Calcium
supplement
p. 123

The mechanisms leading to the loss of bone are still little understood. It is clear that in women after menopause, the increased loss is due to elevated bone resorption following the loss of estrogens, possibly mediated, at least in part, by an increase in IL-6 production. However, it is completely unknown why most people lose bone after a certain age. Various possibilities have been suggested, one of them being a chronic lack of dietary calcium. The amount of calcium which should be ingested is not ← yet completely clear, but it is possible that especially elderly people are deficient in this element. Indeed the aged can also have a vitamin D deficiency due to both a lack of solar exposure and a low dietary intake of vitamin D-containing nutrients. In addition, a disturbance in the metabolism of vitamin D and of its active metabolite $1,25(OH)_2$ vitamin D and of the intestinal receptors of this hormone may induce a decrease in intestinal calcium absorption. This then induces a secondary hyperparathyroidism. It is of interest that in men bone mineral density does not decrease if adjusted for lean body mass. This suggests that the loss might be related to the general atrophy with age, possibly in particular muscle mass, which is then accompanied by a decrease of mechanical forces on the skeleton.

> *While the cause of osteoporosis in postmenopausal women is the lack of estrogens, the cause of the bone loss continuing in the elderly is still unknown. Possibilities are too little calcium in the diet, a low vitamin D status and less mechanical usage.*

→ At the cellular level a discrepancy between bone resorption and formation occurs, the mechanism of which is still unknown. There is a negative balance in each individual element of bone turned over, the BMU, less bone being formed than has been destroyed. The cause after the menopause is an increase in bone resorption, while in the elderly the discrepancy is also caused by a decrease in bone formation, probably because of a decrease in the formation of new osteoblasts. In addition to this imbalance between formation and resorption at the BMU level, estrogen deficiency at the menopause also induces an increase in the number of BMUs formed per unit of time, thus of turnover, which amplifies the total amount of bone lost. In contrast to what was thought previously, the increase in bone turnover is sustained in the elderly. These mechanisms explain why an inhibition of turnover will reduce the bone loss.

BMU
p. 22

Fig. 3.5-5 Mechanisms of bone loss at the microscopic level of the BMU.

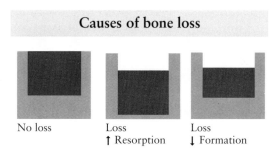

The imbalance lies at the histological level within the individual basic multicellular unit (BMU). This is why an increase in general bone turnover is accompanied by an increase in total bone loss, and why inhibitors of turnover reduce this loss.

3.5.4. Clinical manifestations

Signs and symptoms

The clinical manifestations of osteoporosis are fractures and their consequences. The fractures occur often spontaneously or after minimal trauma. Their location differs somewhat with age. In the postmenopausal form, the forearm is a common site, following a fall on the outstretched hand. Later in life, they occur mostly in the vertebrae, leading to a decrease in height and to forward bending of the spine. This can give rise to nerve compression with pain. In the senile form, hip fractures become increasingly important, both in women and in men. These present a significant morbidity and mortality.

Main osteoporotic fractures			
	Type of fracture		
	Colles'	Vertebral	Hip
Typical age (years)	>55	>65	>75
Women: Men	4:1	3:1	2:1
Predominent bone	Trabecular	Trabecular	Cortical

Fig. 3.5-6 Occurrence of the three typical osteoporotic fractures. (Adapted from the slide kit of the Health Council on Osteoporosis. Reproduced with permission of the author and the publisher).

Although the deterioration in bone mass and possibly architecture is the main cause of the fractures, other factors like a higher propensity to fall and a decreased capacity to handle falls adequately, contribute to their occurrence.

The typical symptom of vertebral osteoporosis is pain, mostly in the back, which can be due to crush fractures or to nerve compression. It has, however, to be remembered that microfractures are usually not accompanied by any acute symptoms, and will only induce a progressive shortening and bending which can then induce chronic back pain.

The main consequence of osteoporosis is fractures. They occur first in the forearm and the spine, later in life in the hip. In the spine, crush fractures can induce pain, shortening and bending and nerve compression.

Laboratory

The investigations to diagnose osteoporosis are radiophysical. Besides plain X-rays to detect fractures, newer techniques such as single energy absorption (SPA and SXA), dual photon absorption (DPA), quantitative computed tomography (QCT) and the now most widely used dual X-ray absorption (DEXA) allow measurement of bone mass. The sites measured are most often the vertebrae, the forearm and the hip.

Osteoporosis is diagnosed and assessed quantitatively by one of the techniques measuring bone mineral density.

Chemical measurements do not permit the diagnosis of osteoporosis *per se*, since they may all be normal. This is especially the case for serum calcium and phosphate and for markers of bone turnover. The latter, assessing bone turnover, are only of use to investigate whether the patient may be in a phase of rapid bone loss. Bone destruction can be evaluated from the urinary levels of hydroxyproline and pyridinoline crosslinks. However, an increase in these values does not necessarily indicate a net loss of bone, since most often bone formation is increased, too, as visualized by elevated levels of serum alkaline phosphatase and osteocalcin. However, if there is a negative balance at the individual BMU, elevated bone turnover will reflect higher bone loss. It should not be forgotten that an elevation of alkaline phosphatase may also indicate the presence of osteomalacia, which is frequently associated with osteoporosis, especially in the old, as well as the presence of a recent fracture.

Assessment of bone turnover p. 27

Chemical analyses such as urinary hydroxyproline and pyridinoline crosslinks or serum alkaline phosphatase cannot be used to diagnose osteoporosis. Most of the time they also cannot be used to evaluate an imbalance between the formation and destruction of bone. They are, however, useful to determine bone turnover and consequently to identify those patients who are likely to be fast bone losers.

Diagnosis

The diagnosis of osteoporosis without complications is made by the quantitative measurement of bone mineral density, that of severe osteoporosis with fractures by X-rays.

Follow-up of evolution

The parameter usually followed in the individual patient is bone mineral density, using one of the techniques able to assess it quantitatively. However, since bone mass changes relatively slowly, measurements are usually not performed more frequently than once every 1–2 years. In the literature it has often been forgotten that many patients, especially the old, also have some degree of osteomalacia. An improvement in bone mineral density may therefore be due to the healing of the osteomalacic component, especially when vitamin D is administered together with another treatment. If bone turnover is high, it is useful to follow the biochemical indices reflecting it, such as urinary hydroxyproline, pyridinoline crosslinks, serum alkaline phosphatase or osteocalcin.

Bone mineral density p. 120

Assessment of bone turnover p. 27

Individual patients are monitored with respect to their bone mineral density, and the chemical parameters of bone turnover. The former reflects the evolution not only of bone mass but also of mineralization. It will therefore also monitor healing of an osteomalacic component.

Although effects on fracture rates are likely to parallel those of bone density, it will nevertheless be necessary in the future, when assessing new treatments, to determine whether they are accompanied at least by an amelioration of the mechanical properties in the animal, or better by a decrease in fracture incidence in humans. However, the number of patients necessary to achieve statistical significance for the latter is very large.

3.5.5. Treatment with drugs other than bisphosphonates

In general, treatments can be divided into two categories, namely those aiming at the inhibition of loss or further loss of bone, and those aiming to increase bone mass.

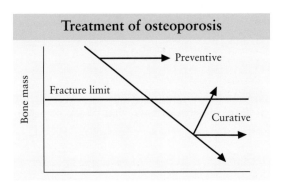

Fig. 3.5-7 Preventive and curative treatment of osteoporosis.

Treatment of osteoporosis can be both preventive and curative.

Some treatments are available that inhibit bone destruction and therefore prevent future or further bone loss. The most widely used is estrogen replacement after the menopause. This treatment is very effective in inhibiting bone loss and even leads to a small increase in bone density. Moreover, it greatly reduces the occurrence of fractures of the wrist, hip and spine. Many women, however, refuse this therapy for various reasons, not the least being the fear of a possible slight increase in the frequency of breast cancer. However, there seems to be no increase in breast cancer mortality in estrogen-treated women. The increased risk of endometrial carcinoma can be completely prevented by the simultaneous administration of a progestagen. Estrogens also reduce the risk of cardiovascular disease, which otherwise rises after the menopause, and improve urogenital symptoms. One current approach consists in developing partial estrogen agonists, retaining the effects on bone and lipids, but devoid of effects on other tissues. Statistical evaluation of all the risks is currently in progress in large studies.

Fig. 3.5-8 Effect of estrogen and gestagen on bone loss. (Adapted from Christiansen, C. *et al.* (1981). Reproduced with permission from the author and the publisher.)

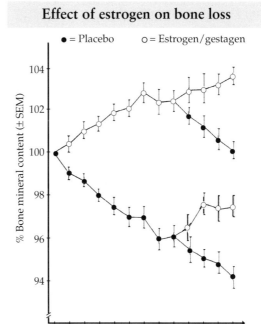

The other drug that inhibits bone resorption and decreases bone loss is calcitonin. The main problems of this treatment has been the sometimes unpleasant side effects and the necessity of frequent subcutaneous administration. These disadvantages appear to be solved to a large extent with the recent availability of nasal preparations.

Calcium can also decrease bone loss in certain conditions. Many of the recent studies indicate that it decreases bone turnover. It finds its use mostly in the elderly and possibly in the growing child and adolescent. Today it is thought that in women a daily intake of 1 g in the adult, more

Dietary calcium p. 25

in adolescents, during lactation and in the elderly, is required. No information is available for men. Furthermore, calcium supplementation of at least 500 mg daily is a standard procedure when either an inhibitor of bone resorption or a stimulator of formation is given. Vitamin D should be present in sufficient amounts. Recently it was shown that the administration of 1 g of calcium and 800 units of vitamin D to elderly institutionalized women decreased the rate of hip and other non-vertebral fractures. How much of this improvement was due to the presence of osteomalacia is not known. Also, $1,25(OH)_2$ vitamin D can decrease bone loss in certain patients, especially in Japan, but the benefit over vitamin D is still controversial.

The most suitable preventive treatment of osteoporosis in women at risk after the menopause is estrogen. If estrogen treatment is not possible, this might be replaced by calcium and calcitonin. In elderly people, calcium together with vitamin D, especially if they are vitamin D deficient, is the therapy of choice and reduces the fracture rate.

Today only very few compounds are able to increase bone formation, namely fluoride and PTH. Fluoride administered as sodium fluoride or monofluorophosphate increases cancellous bone, the effect on the cortex being less clear. A regimen of 75 mg of sodium fluoride per day, equal to 34 mg of fluoride ion, for 4 years has led to no change in vertebral fractures, but possibly to an increase in non-vertebral fractures. This dosage also gives rise to unpleasant adverse events, such as bone pain due to microfractures, a consequence of an inhibition of mineralization, and to gastrointestinal disturbances. However, lower doses of 15–25 mg fluoride ion daily still increase bone mass, decrease vertebral fractures but do not increase non-vertebral fractures, and give rise to much fewer adverse events especially if administered in a slow-release form. A multicenter study of the effects at this lower dosage is in progress. PTH is still under clinical investigation.

Only fluoride and PTH are able to increase bone formation. Fluoride appears to decrease vertebral fractures, but its effect on hip fractures is not yet clear. The safety margin of this drug is relatively narrow.

3.5.6. Treatment with bisphosphonates

Preclinical studies

→ Many animal experiments support the use of bisphosphonates in humans. As described earlier, in normal growing rats these compounds decrease bone resorption and increase calcium balance and the mineral content of bone.

Rat studies
pp. 39–43

Effect on
Ca balance
p. 42

Besides actually increasing bone mass in normal animals, the bisphosphonates are also effective in preventing bone loss in a number of experimental osteoporosis models. The first used was immobilization by sciatic nerve section in the rat.

Fig. 3.5-9 Effect of 10 mg P/kg of clodronate subcutaneously on the bone loss induced by sciatic nerve section in the rat.
(Data from Mühlbauer, R.C. *et al.* (1971).)

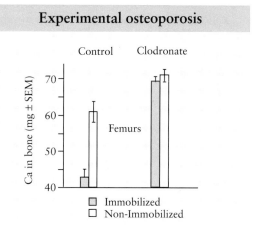

Later, similar results were obtained in a number of osteoporosis models not only in the rat, but also in the mouse, rabbit, dog and monkey.

Fig. 3.5-10 Osteoporosis models improved by bisphosphonates.

Osteoporosis models

- Sciatic nerve section
- Paraplegia
- Hypokinesia
- Ovariectomy
- Orchidectomy
- Heparin
- Thyroid hormones
- Corticosteroids
- Low calcium

Practically all the bisphosphonates tested, such as, in order of increasing potency, etidronate, tiludronate, clodronate, pamidronate, olpadronate, cimadronate, alendronate, risedronate, ibandronate and YH 529, have been effective. In the case of etidronate, the effect was blurred when

Chemical
structures
pp. 35–36

higher doses were used which inhibited mineralization. In the ovariectomized rat the preventive effect was maintained for a long period after discontinuation of the drug.

Bisphosphonates prevent bone loss in practically all the experimental osteoporosis models.

The question of the effect of the bisphosphonates upon the mechanical properties of the skeleton has been addressed only recently. This issue is of importance, since it is known that a long-lasting, strong inhibition of bone resorption can lead to increased bone fragility both in animals and in humans, the human osteopetrosis described by Albers–Schönberg being a good illustration. It appears that, when not given in excess, bisphosphonates have a positive effect on mechanical characteristics both in normal animals and in various experimental osteoporosis models. The bisphosphonates that proved to be active include etidronate, although at high doses the opposite effect was induced, probably because of an inhibition of mineralization, alendronate, cimadronate, clodronate, neridronate, olpadronate, pamidronate, tiludronate and YH 529.

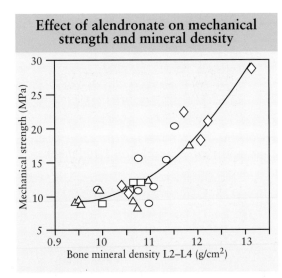

Effect of alendronate on mechanical strength and mineral density

Fig. 3.5-11 Effect of alendronate given intravenously every 2 weeks for a period of 2 years to ovariectomized baboons on bone mineral density and mechanical strength. Squares, not ovariectomized; triangles, ovariectomized; circles, ovariectomized + 0.05 mg/kg; diamonds, ovariectomized + 0.25 mg/kg; MPa, megapascal. (Adapted from Balena, R. *et al.* (1993). Reproduced from *J. Clin. Invest.*, **92**, 2577–86, with copyright permission from the author and the American Society of Clinical Investigation.)

The bisphosphonates can, by increasing bone mass, improve the mechanical strength of the bones both in normal animals and in those with experimental osteoporosis.

The mechanism of action of the bisphosphonates in osteoporosis is still not completely understood. The prevention of bone loss is probably explained to a large extent by the decrease in bone turnover which slows down bone loss. This decrease also diminishes the fracture rate, since fewer trabeculae are destroyed. In addition, the bisphosphonates also act at the individual BMU by decreasing the depth of the resorption site.

Mechanisms of bone loss p. 119

→ The actual increase in bone mass which is sometimes seen, probably has various causes. One explanation of this increase is that the decrease in bone resorption is followed only later by the 'coupling-induced' diminution in formation, which brings a temporary gain in calcium balance through the reduction of the so-called remodeling space. Another interesting possibility is that by lowering resorption less than formation at the individual BMU level, the bisphosphonates increase bone balance at this site. Such an effect has been demonstrated in man.

Coupling pp. 22–23

BMU p. 22

Effect in man p. 131

→ Fig. 3.5-12 Possible effect of bisphosphonates at the level of the individual BMU.

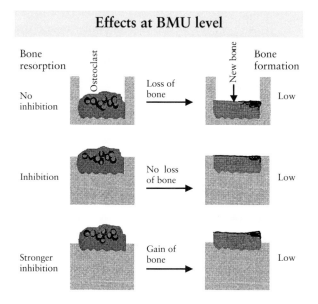

Effects at BMU level

Bone resorption — Osteoclast

No inhibition — Loss of bone → New bone — Bone formation — Low

Inhibition — No loss of bone → Low

Stronger inhibition — Gain of bone → Low

→ Finally, it has recently been suggested that alendronate to some extent increases bone formation at the level of the BMU in OVX baboons. A similar effect has been suggested in humans with clodronate. If these findings are confirmed, it could be concluded that bisphosphonates could also act by increasing bone formation, which has always been negated until now.

Effect of formation *in vitro* p. 53

Bisphosphonates act in osteoporosis by decreasing turnover and possibly changing the balance at the level of the individual bone multicellular unit (BMU).

Of clinical importance is the recent finding that treatments which increase bone formation, such as prostaglandin, IGF-I and PTH, are still effective in rats treated by bisphosphonates, resulting in an additive effect of the two treatments. One study on sheep showed, however, the loss of $1,25(OH)_2$-induced increase in osteocalcin under bisphosphonate administration.

Clinical studies ←

Effects

While there have been quite a number of studies using bisphosphonates in patients with osteoporosis, there were until recently only few that were adequately controlled. The many uncontrolled studies suggest, however, that various bisphosphonates would not only stop the loss of bone in postmenopausal osteoporosis and other types of the disease, but would actually induce a small increase in bone mineral density.

A series of studies, although inadequately controlled, suggested that various bisphosphonates not only slow down or stop bone loss, but can actually induce an increase in bone mineral density.

The first controlled study was performed in the 1970s with etidronate at an oral dose of 20 mg/kg daily for 6 months in senile osteoporosis. The results were not very encouraging, since bone resorption and formation decreased approximately to the same extent, so that the effect on calcium balance was only small. However, at the above dose and regimen an inhibition of mineralization was, in the opinion of the author, likely to have occurred. Thus, a positive bone balance, if present, would have been obscured.

Inhibition of mineralization pp. 148–150

More recently, various controlled studies showed that bisphosphonates can indeed stop bone loss in osteoporosis. Two controlled double-blind studies investigated the effect in postmenopausal women of discontinuous oral administration of etidronate for 2 weeks, followed in both the etidronate and the placebo groups by either 10 or 13 weeks of 500 mg daily of calcium. The cycle was repeated over a period of 3 years and in some patients up to 4 years more. Both studies showed a small but significant increase of vertebral bone mineral content, in contrast to a loss in one study, and no change in the other (*see* Fig. 3.5-13). Some increase in mineral was still observed between 5 and 7 years of treatment. Similar results were also obtained in the hip (*see* Fig. 3.5-14). Recent data showed that etidronate is also effective in preventing bone loss in non-osteoporotic women just after the menopause.

Fig. 3.5-13 Effect of etidronate administered for 2 weeks every 3 months for 4 years on bone mineral density in postmenopausal osteo-porosis. In the first 3 years the study was double-blind, in the last year all patients received etidronate. (Adapted from Harris, S.T. *et al.* (1993). Reproduced from the *J. Med.*, **95**, 557–67, with permission from the author and the publisher.)

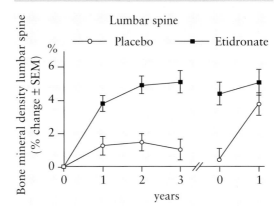

Fig. 3.5-14 Effect of etidronate adminis-tered for 3 years on the bone mineral density of the hip. The study was the same as in Fig. 3.5-13. (Adapted from Harris, S.T. *et al.* (1993). Reproduced from the *J. Med.*, **95**, 557–67, with permis-sion from the author and publisher.)

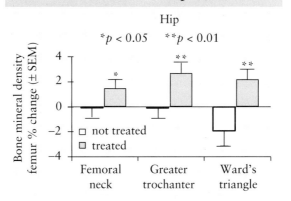

Histogical investigations showed that at the level of the BMU the bis-phosphonate induced a decrease in bone turnover, a decrease in the depth of the resorptive cavities and no change or possibly an increase in the amount of new bone formed. The results may in part explain the in-crease in bone density.

BMU
p. 127

Of interest is the recent finding that after long-term (between 4 and 7 years) intermittent therapy with etidronate as described above, bone turnover rates assessed histologically returned towards baseline, although bone mineral density did not decrease. If confirmed also with biochemical markers of bone turnover, this result would allay the con-cern that long-term bisphosphonate therapy diminishes turnover to an extent which may be associated with increased skeletal fragility.

Similar results on bone mineral density were also found with tiludronate administered for 6 months and with clodronate given one month
out of three for 1 year. In the first study, the effect was apparently maintained over 2 years, the duration of the study, despite discontinuation of
the drug. Similar effects on bone density have also been observed with
pamidronate given orally for 2 years or intravenously once every 3
months.

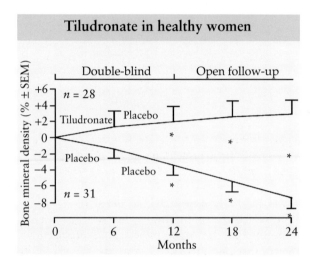

Fig. 3.5-15 Effect of 6-month oral treatment with 100 mg tiludronate on lumbar bone mineral density of healthy postmenopausal women; $p < 0.01$. (Adapted from Reginster, J.Y. (1992). *Bone*, **13**, 351–4. Reproduced with permission from the author and publisher.)

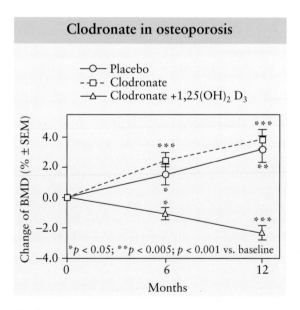

Fig. 3.5-16 Effect of clodronate adminis-tered at 400 mg/day for 30 days every 3 months in post-menopausal women. □ clodronate; △ 2 µg/day $1,25(OH)_2$ vitamin D_3 for 5 days and clodronate for 25 days; ○ placebo. (Adapted from Giannini, S. *et al.* (1993). Reproduced from *Bone*, **14**, 137–41, with copyright permission from the author and Elsevier Science Ltd., The Boulevard, Langhford Lane, Kidlington OX5 IGB, UK.)

Fig. 3.5-17 Effect of a 2-year oral treatment with 150 mg pamidronate daily on the lumbar spine density of patients with postmenopausal osteoporosis. (Adapted from Reid, I.R. *et al.* (1994) *J. Clin. Endocrinol. Metab*, 79, 1595–9, with permission from the author and publisher.)

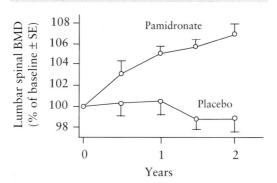

Clodronate, etidronate, tiludronate and pamidronate not only prevent the decrease in bone mass in postmenopausal osteoporosis, but actually induce a small increase in bone mineral content.

Recently various studies have demonstrated that alendronate is also effective in this regard. In the first study the compound was given intravenously every 3 months. In the other two studies, both multicentric, randomized and placebo controlled, the administration was given orally at 5 mg, 10 mg, 20 mg and 40 mg for 2 years. All the studies have shown

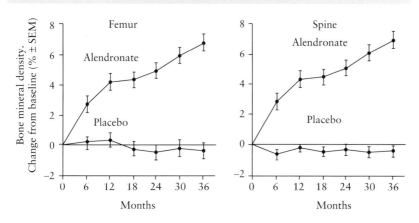

Fig. 3.5-18 Effect of 10 mg alendronate given daily for 3 years on bone mineral density of the hip and the spine in patients with postmenopausal osteoporosis. (Courtesy of Merck Research Laboratories, USA.)

an increase in bone density both in the vertebrae and in the hip, compared with a drop or no change in the controls. Since 10 mg were more active than 5 mg, but not less active than 20 mg, 10 mg appears to be the most favorable dose. A 3-year study showed similar results, with an increase of about 7% compared with a loss of about 1%. A plateau seems to have been reached after 2 years in the spine, but not in the hip.

> *Alendronate administered orally at 10 mg per day for 3 years induced a 7% increase of bone mineral density in the spine and the hip, compared with a 1% loss in the controls.*

Iliac bone biopsies in over 200 patients have shown that three parameters of mineralization, namely osteoid thickness, osteoid volume and mineral apposition rate were normal even at a daily dose of 20 mg for 2 years. This shows that at this dosage no inhibition of mineralization has occurred. In all the biopsies the new bone was lamellar, without any signs of cell toxicity.

Effects in rat
p. 59
It is interesting that in analogy to what has been seen in rats and ← baboons, the inhibitory effect on bone destruction reaches a plateau even if the administration is continued, and that this plateau is dependent on the dose administered. With appropriate dosage, premenopausal levels can be reached. Furthermore the inhibition of resorption disappears when the drug is discontinued. These results suggest that the bisphosphonate buried in the bone is inactive, and that there is no danger of a continuous decrease of bone turnover with an increase in bone fragility.

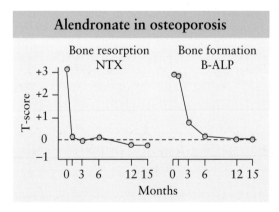

Fig. 3.5-19 Effect of alendronate on bone turnover assessed by the urinary excretion of crosslinked N-telopeptides (NTX) and serum alkaline phosphatase (B-ALP) in patients with postmenopausal osteoporosis. The plateau reached corresponds to the premenopausal levels. T-score = 1 SD from the latter values. (Adapted from Garnero, P. *et al.* (1994). Reproduced with the permission from the author and the publisher.)

> *The inhibition of bone resorption reaches a plateau which is dependent of the dosage, even if the administration is continued.*

Recent results show that alendronate and etidronate are also effective in healthy postmenopausal women and that alendronate is effective in 70–80 year-old women. Finally, risedronate at daily oral doses of 5 mg given for up to 2 years induced a higher bone mass than placebo.

The question of whether bisphosphonates will also decrease fracture incidence was open, until very recently. Some decrease in vertebral fractures was found in both etidronate studies, but the significance of this result is still not clearly established.

Fig. 3.5-20   Effect of etidronate administered for 2 weeks every 3 months for 3 years on vertebral fractures. In the left panel all patients were included, while in the right only those with a low bone mineral density at the start were analyzed (Adapted from Harris, S.T. *et al.* (1993). Reproduced from *J. Med.*, 95, 557–67, with permission from the author and publisher.)

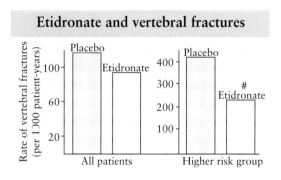

The effect of etidronate on fracture rate looks promising but is not yet clear and needs further investigation.

Just when this book went into press, it was reported that the daily oral administration of 10 mg of alendronate for 3 years to over 900 postmenopausal osteoporotic women led to a decrease of 48% in vertebral fractures. In addition, also non-vertebral fractures were decreased significantly.

Alendronate given orally for 3 years decreases by half the occurrence of vertebral fractures and decreases also non-vertebral fractures.

Some data are also available in other types of osteoporosis. Clodronate decreased bone loss in paraplegia; etidronate and pamidronate inhibited both metacarpal and vertebral loss induced by corticosteroid therapy.

Treatment regimens

Alendronate

Commercially
available
bisphosphonates
pp. 157–170

In the first published study 5 mg intravenously every 3 months was used. Later, daily oral doses between 5 and 40 mg were given. All regimens have been effective in increasing bone density. Today 10 mg daily given continuously orally is the regimen suggested by the producer. Alendronate is registered in various countries.

Clodronate

The first published controlled study was performed in paraplegia where daily oral doses of 400 and 1600 mg given continuously somewhat diminished the bone loss. More recently 400 mg were daily given orally for one month out of three for 1 year. To our knowledge, clodronate so far is registered for osteoporosis only in Italy. The recommended regimen is 400 mg daily for 1 month every 3 months, or the same dose continuously.

Etidronate

Inhibition of
mineralization
pp. 148–150

Up to now, the only dosage which has been adequately studied is discontinuous treatment with 400 mg daily orally for 14 days, followed by 10 or 13 weeks without drug. All patients received a supplement of 500 mg of calcium daily. This regimen was effective in stopping bone loss, and at this dose the drug appears to be very safe, at least for up to 4 years. Whether this is the case also after a longer treatment with this regimen is not yet certain, since in one of the studies there were some signs of focal abnormalities of mineralization after 4–5 years of therapy. However, it is not known whether these changes have any clinical relevance. Furthermore, no signs of more generalized osteomalacia were seen even after 7 years of treatment.

So far it is not known whether another regimen would give better results. A higher dosage should, however, not be used, since an inhibition of mineralization may occur. It is also not known whether it might be preferable to interrupt treatment from time to time.

Commercially
available
bisphosphonates
pp. 157–170

Etidronate is commercially available in many countries for this indication.

The recommended regimen for etidronate is 400 mg daily orally for 2 weeks every 3 months. How long such a treatment should be pursued without interruption is not yet determined.

Pamidronate

In steroid-induced osteoporosis, pamidronate was effective at an oral daily dose of 150 mg for 1 year. In other non-controlled studies, this dose also appeared effective. The same dose was also effective in increasing bone mass in postmenopausal osteoporosis. The same was true for the intravenous administration of 30 mg every 3 months. To our knowledge, pamidronate is registered for osteoporosis only in Argentina and Uruguay.

Commercially available bisphosphonates pp. 157–170

Tiludronate

The only dosage tested was an oral dose of 100 mg daily for 6 months. Tiludronate is not registered in any country for osteoporosis.

Conclusion

Bisphosphonates not only stop bone loss in various types of osteoporosis, but even induce a small increase in bone mineral density. At least alendronate decreases vertebral fractures. These compounds are likely to become an important addition to the therapeutic modalities available for the prevention and possibly the treatment of osteoporosis.

Recommended selected reading

Osteoporosis

Books

Christiansen, C. and Riis, B. (1990). *The Silent Epidemic. Post-Menopausal Osteoporosis.* Christiansen, C. and Riis, B., Fagerstien 8, 2950 Vedbaek, Denmark

Kanis, J.A. (1994). *Osteoporosis.* (Oxford: Blackwell Science)

Riggs, B.L. and Melton, L.J. III (eds.) (1988). *Osteoporosis. Etiology, Diagnosis, and Management.* (New York: Raven Press)

WHO Study Group (1994). *Assessment of Fracture Risk and its Application to Screening for Postmenopausal Osteoporosis.* WHO Technical Report Series, 843. (Geneva: World Health Organization)

Reviews

Dunn, C.J., Fitton, A. and Sorkin, E.M. (1994). Etidronic acid. A review of its pharmaco-logical properties and therapeutic efficacy in resorptive bone disease. *Drugs Aging*, 5, 446–74

Christiansen, C. (ed.) (1993). *Proceedings of the Consensus Development Conference on Osteoporosis*, Hong Kong, April 1–2. *Am. J. Med.*, 95 (Suppl. 5A), 1S–78S

Consensus development conference (1993). Diagnosis, prophylaxis and treatment of osteo-porosis. *Am. J. Med.*, 94, 646–50

Eriksen, E.F. and Mosekilde, L. (1990). Estrogens and bone. In Heersche, J.N.M. and Kanis, J.A. (eds.) *Bone and Mineral Research*, vol. 7, pp. 273–312. (Amsterdam, New York, Oxford: Elsevier)

Gruber, H.E. and Baylink, D.J. (1991). The effects of fluoride on bone. *Clin. Orthop.*, 267, 264–77

Jackson, J.A. and Kleerekoper, M. (1990). Osteoporosis in men: diagnosis, pathophysi-ology, and prevention. *Medicine (Baltimore)*, 69, 137–52

Lindsay, R. and Cosman, F. (1992). Primary osteoporosis. In Coe, F.L. and Favus, M.J. (eds.) *Disorders of Bone and Mineral Metabolism*, pp. 831–88. (New York: Raven Press)

Marcus, R. (1992). Secondary forms of osteoporosis. In Coe, F.L. and Favus, M.J. (eds.) *Disorders of Bone and Mineral Metabolism*, pp. 889–904. (New York: Raven Press)

Raisz, L.G. and Shourki, K.C. (1993). Pathogenesis of osteoporosis. In Mundy, G.R. and Martin, T.J. (eds.) *Physiology and Pharmacology of Bone. Handbook of Experimental Pharmacology*, vol. 107, pp. 299–331

Riggs, B.L. and Melton, L.J. III (1986). Involution osteoporosis. *N. Engl. J. Med.*, 314, 1676–86

Riggs, B.L. and Melton, L.J. III (1992). The prevention and treatment of osteoporosis. *N. Engl. J. Med.*, 327, 620–7

Bisphosphonates, general

Reviews

Dunn, C.J., Fitton, A. and Sorkin, E.M. (1994). Etidronic acid. A review of its pharmaco-logical properties and therapeutic efficacy in resorptive bone disease. *Drugs Aging*, 5, 446–74

Fleisch, H. (1993). Bisphosphonates: mechanisms of action and clinical use. In Mundy, G.R. and Martin, T.J. (eds.) *Physiology and Pharmacology of Bone*, pp. 377–418. (Berlin, Heidelberg, New York: Springer-Verlag)

Papapoulos, S.E., Landman, J.O., Bijvoet, O.L.M., Löwik, C.W.G.M., Valkema, R., Pauwels, E.K.J. and Vermeij, P. (1992). The use of bisphosphonates in the treatment of osteoporosis. *Bone*, 13 (Suppl.1), S41–S49

Original articles

Bisphosphonates, preclinical

Ammann, P., Rizzoli, R., Caverzasio, J., Shigematsu, T., Slosman, D. and Bonjour, J.P. (1993). Effects of the bisphosphonate tiludronate on bone resorption, calcium balance, and bone mineral density. *J. Bone Miner. Res.*, 8, 1491–8

Balena, R., Toolan, B.C., Shea, M., Markatos, A., Myers, E.R., Lee, S.C., Opas, E.E., Seedor, J.G., Klein, H., Frankenfield, D., Quartuccio, H., Fioravanti, C., Clair, J., Brown, E., Hayes, W.C. and Rodan, G.A. (1993). The effects of 2-year treatment with the aminobisphosphonate alendronate on bone metabolism, bone histomorphometry, and bone strength in ovariectomized nonhuman primates. *J. Clin. Invest.*, **92**, 2577–86

Ferretti, J.L., Delgado, C.J., Capozza, R.F., Cointry, G., Montuori, E., Roldán, E., Pérez Lloret, A. and Zanchetta, J.R. (1993). Protective effects of disodium etidronate and pamidronate against the biomechanical repercussion of betamethasone-induced osteopenia in growing rat femurs. *Bone Miner.*, **20**, 265–76

Jee, W.S.S., Black, H.E. and Gotcher, J.E. (1981). Effect of dichloromethane diphosphonate on cortisol-induced bone loss in young adult rabbits. *Clin. Orthop.*, **156**, 39–51

Monier-Faugere, M-C., Friedler, R.M., Bauss, F. and Malluche, H.H. (1993). A new bisphosphonate, BM 21.0955, prevents bone loss associated with cessation of ovarian function in experimental dogs. *J. Bone Min. Res.*, **8**, 1345–55

Motoie, H., Nakamura, T., O'Uchi, N., Nishikawa, H., Kanoh, H., Abe, T. and Kawashima, H. (1995). Effects of the bisphosphonate YM175 on bone mineral density, strength, structure, and turnover in ovariectomized beagles on concomitant dietary calcium restriction. *J. Bone Miner. Res.*, **10**, 910–20

Mühlbauer, R.C., Russell, R.G.G., Williams, D.A. and Fleisch, H. (1971). The effects of diphosphonates, polyphosphates, and calcitonin on 'immobilisation' osteoporosis in rats. *Eur. J. Clin. Invest.*, **1**, 336–44

Murakami, H., Nakamura, T., Tsurukami, H., Abe, M., Barbier, A. and Suzuki, K. (1994). Effects of tiludronate on bone mass, structure, and turnover at the epiphyseal, primary, and secondary spongiosa in the proximal tibia of growing rats after sciatic neurectomy. *J. Bone Miner. Res.*, **9**, 1355–64

Rosen, H.N., Sullivan, E.K., Middlebrooks, V.L., Zeind, A.J., Gundberg, C., Dresner-Pollak, R., Maitland, L.A., Hock, J.M., Moses, A.C. and Greenspan, S.L. (1993). Parenteral pamidronate prevents thyroid hormone induced bone loss in rats. *J. Bone Miner. Res.*, **8**, 1255–61

Thompson, D.D., Seedor, J.G., Quartuccio, H., Solomon, H., Fioravanti, C., Davidson, J., Klein, H., Jackson, R., Clair, J., Frankenfield, D., Brown, E., Simmons, H.A. and Rodan, G.A. (1992). The bisphosphonate, alendronate, prevents bone loss in ovariectomized baboons. *J. Bone Miner. Res.*, **7**, 951–60

Toolan, B.C., Shea, M., Myers, E.R., Borchers, R.E., Seedor, J.G., Quartuccio, H., Rodan, G. and Hayes, W.C. (1992). Effects of 4-amino-1-hydroxybutylidene bisphosphonate on bone biomechanics in rats. *J. Bone Miner. Res.*, **7**, 1399–406

Wronski, T.J., Dann, L.M., Qi, H. and Yen, C.F. (1993). Skeletal effects of withdrawal of estrogen and diphosphonate treatment in ovariectomized rats. *Calcif. Tissue Int.*, **53**, 210–16

Bisphosphonates, clinical

Alendronate

Adami, S., Baroni, M.C., Broggini, M., Carratelli, L., Caruso, I., Gnessi, L., Laurenzi, M., Lombardi, A., Norbiato, G., Ortolani, S., Ricerca, E., Romanini, L., Subrizi, S., Weinberg, J. and Yates, A.J. (1993). Treatment of postmenopausal osteoporosis with continuous daily oral alendronate in comparison with either placebo or intranasal salmon calcitonin. *Osteoporosis Int.* (Suppl. 3), S21–S27

Osteoporosis

Chesnut, C.H. III, McClung, M.R., Ensrud, K.E., Bell, N.H., Genant, H.K., Harris, S.T., Singer, F.R., Stock, J.L., Yood, R.L., Delmas, P.D., Kher, U., Pryor-Tillotson, S. and Santora, A.C. II (1995). Alendronate treatment of the postmenopausal osteoporotic woman: effect of multiple dosages on bone mass and bone remodeling. *Am. J. Med.*, **99**,144–52

Garnero, P., Shih, W.J., Gineyts, E., Karpf, D.B. and Delmas, P.D. (1994). Comparison of new biochemical markers of bone turnover in late postmenopausal osteoporotic women in response to alendronate treatment. *J. Clin. Endocrinol. Metab.*, **79**, 1693–700

Gertz, B.J., Shao, P., Hanson, D.A., Quan, H., Harris, S.T., Genant, H.K., Chesnut, C.H. III and Eyre, D.R. (1994). Monitoring bone resorption in early postmenopausal women by an immunoassay for cross-linked collagen peptides in urine. *J. Bone Miner. Res.*, **9**, 135–42

Passeri, M., Baroni, M.C., Pedrazzoni, M., Pioli, G., Barbagallo, M., Costi, D., Biondi, M., Girasole, G., Arlunno, B. and Palummeri, E. (1991). Intermittent treatment with intravenous 4-amino-1-hydroxybutylidene-1,1-bisphosphonate (AHBuBP) in the therapy of postmenopausal osteoporosis. *Bone Miner.*, **15**, 237–47

Clodronate

Giannini, S., D'Angelo, A., Malvasi, L., Castrignano, R., Pati, T., Tronca, R., Liberto, L., Nobile, M. and Crepaldi, G. (1993). Effects of one-year cyclical treatment with clodronate on postmenopausal bone loss. *Bone*, **14**, 137–41

Minaire, P., Bérard, E., Meunier, P.J., Edouard, C., Goedert, G. and Pilonchéry, G. (1981). Effects of disodium dichloromethylene diphosphonate on bone loss in paraplegic patients. *J. Clin. Invest.*, **68**, 1086–92

Etidronate

Harris, S.T., Watts, N.B., Jackson, R.D., Genant, H.K., Wasnich, R.D., Ross, P., Miller, P.D., Licata, A.A. and Chesnut, C.H. III (1993). Four-year study of intermittent cyclic etidronate treatment of postmenopausal osteoporosis: three years of blinded therapy followed by one year of open therapy. *Am. J. Med.*, **95**, 557–67

Heaney, R.P. and Saville, P.D. (1976). Etidronate disodium in postmenopausal osteoporosis. *Clin. Pharmacol. Ther.*, **20**, 593–604

Storm, T., Steiniche, T., Thamsborg, G. and Melsen, F. (1993). Changes in bone histomorphometry after long-term treatment with intermittent, cyclic etidronate for postmenopausal osteoporosis. *J. Bone Miner. Res.*, **8**, 199–208

Storm, T., Thamsborg, G., Steiniche, T., Genant, H.K. and Sorensen, O.H. (1990). Effect of intermittent cyclical etidronate therapy on bone mass and fracture rate in women with postmenopausal osteoporosis. *N. Engl. J. Med.*, **322**, 1265–71

Watts, N.B., Harris, S.T., Genant, H.K., Wasnich, R.D., Miller, P.D., Jackson, R.D., Licata, A.A., Ross, P., Woodson, G.C., Yanover, M.J., Mysiw, W.J., Kohse, L., Rao, M.B., Steiger, P., Richmond, B. and Chesnut, C.H. III (1990). Intermittent cyclical etidronate treatment of postmenopausal osteoporosis. *N. Engl. J. Med.*, **323**, 73–9

Pamidronate

Reid, I.R., King, A.R., Alexander, C.J. and Ibbertson, H.K. (1988). Prevention of steroid-induced osteoporosis with (3-amino-1-hydroxypropylidene)-1,1-bisphosphonate (APD). *Lancet*, **1**, 143–6

Reid, I.R., Wattie, D.J., Evans, M.C., Gamble, G.D., Stapleton, J.P. and Cornish, J. (1994). Continuous therapy with pamidronate, a potent bisphosphonate, in postmenopausal osteoporosis. *J. Clin. Endocrinol. Metab.*, **79**, 1595–9

Thiébaud, D., Burckhardt, P., Melchior, J., Eckert, P., Jacquet, A.F., Schnyder, P. and Gobelet, C. (1994). Two years' effectiveness of intravenous pamidronate (APD) versus oral fluoride for osteoporosis occurring in the postmenopause. *Osteoporosis Int.*, **4**, 76–83

Valkema, R., Vismans, F.J.F.E., Papapoulos, S.E., Pauwels, E.K.J. and Bijvoet, O.L.M. (1989). Maintained improvement in calcium balance and bone mineral content in patients with osteoporosis treated with the bisphosphonate APD. *Bone Miner.*, **5**, 183–92

Tiludronate

Chappard, D., Minaire, P., Privat, C., Bérard, E., Mendoza-Sarmiento, J., Tournebise, H., Basle, M.F., Audran, M., Rebel, A., Picot, C. and Gaud, C. (1995). Effects of tiludronate on bone loss in paraplegic patients. *J. Bone Miner. Res.*, **10**, 112–8

Reginster, J.Y., Lecart, M.P., Deroisy, R., Sarlet, N., Denis, D., Ethgen, D., Collette, J. and Franchimont, P. (1989). Prevention of postmenopausal bone loss by tiludronate. *Lancet*, **2**, 1469–71

3.6. HETEROTOPIC CALCIFICATION AND OSSIFICATION

3.6.1. Definition

Heterotopic, also called ectopic, calcification is a condition in which calcium phosphate deposits in sites that are normally not calcified. If the calcification occurs in the form of osseous or osseous-like tissue, the condition is called heterotopic ossification.

A distinction is made between heterotopic calcification and heterotopic ossification.

3.6.2. Pathophysiology

Ectopic calcification can occur in various tissues. Its mechanism is not understood, except when it occurs during hypercalcemia or in the case of urinary stones. In these cases precipitation occurs, because of the supersaturation of the fluid in calcium and phosphate. Local disturbances of nucleators or of inhibitors of calcium phosphate crystal formation are an attractive hypothesis.

The cause of heterotopic ossification is unknown. Here the abnormal formation of bone usually occurs in the muscles and trauma seems to be involved in some cases. Heterotopic ossification is common after hip operations with implantation of a prosthesis, after paraplegia and after cerebral trauma. In other cases, such as fibrodysplasia ossificans progressiva, the disorder is congenital. Possibly an imbalance of local growth factors, such as the bone morphogenetic proteins, could be involved.

The mechanisms responsible for the development of the heterotopic calcifications and ossifications are unknown.

3.6.3. Clinical manifestations

Manifestations are numerous and depend upon the localization of the calcium phosphate deposit. In the case of heterotopic calcification, the most frequent location is in the walls of blood vessels, especially the arteries. In the lumen of the urinary tract, they will lead to the formation of urolithiasis. Calcification can be widespread throughout the connective tissues in conditions such as calcinosis universalis, dermatomyositis and scleroderma.

Heterotopic ossification can be localized, for example after hip prosthesis, or widespread, as in fibrodysplasia ossificans progressiva, where death as a result of pulmonary insufficiency can occur.

3.6.4. Treatment with drugs other than bisphosphonates

Many therapies have been tried in heterotopic calcification, but none has proven totally successful. In heterotopic ossification, for example after hip replacement, the treatments most often used are non-steroidal anti-inflammatory agents and irradiation.

3.6.5. Treatment with bisphosphonates

The only bisphosphonate investigated up to now is etidronate.

Preclinical studies

As mentioned earlier, bisphosphonates very efficiently inhibit mineralization *in vivo*. They can prevent experimentally induced calcification of many soft tissues such as arteries, kidneys, skin, heart, heart valves, urinary stones when given parenterally or orally and, when administered topically, experimental dental calculus. Etidronate also inhibits ectopic ossification induced by various means.

Action on calcification pp. 50–51

> **Bisphosphonates prevent experimental heterotopic calcification and ossification in animals.**

Clinical studies

The studies mentioned above led to the hope that bisphosphonates would find a use in preventing ectopic calcification and ossification in humans. Unfortunately, the results obtained so far are less encouraging than expected. The studies all used etidronate, which is therefore the only bisphosphonate investigated so far. They were usually uncontrolled and performed on only very few patients in diseases that undergo spontaneous remission, so that the results are difficult to interpret.

Heterotopic calcification

Soft tissue calcification

Etidronate has been given in some cases of scleroderma, dermatomyositis, idiopathic infantile arterial calcification and calcinosis universalis. Efficacy is uncertain, since these disorders often go into spontaneous remission.

The efficacy of etidronate in various ectopic soft tissue calcifications is uncertain.

Urolithiasis

Physicochemical effects p. 38

The hope that the inhibitory effect on crystal growth and aggregation of both calcium phosphate and calcium oxalate would be useful for the prevention of urinary stones has not been fulfilled, at least with etidronate. Although pilot studies showed an effect in chronic stone formers, the dose necessary to obtain inhibition of crystal growth in urine was high, about 1600 mg/day orally, so that it would also induce inhibition of skeletal mineralization. Furthermore, the clinical benefit is uncertain, large scale studies having failed to show efficacy. Etidronate can therefore not be recommended for use in urolithiasis.

Adverse events pp. 148–150

Etidronate should not be administered in urolithiasis.

Dental calculus

Many investigations have shown that topical application of etidronate by means of mouthwashes or toothpastes diminishes the development of dental calculus. A toothpaste containing a bisphosphonate is marketed in some countries.

A bisphosphonate is commercially available in a toothpaste against dental calculus.

Heterotopic ossification

Fibrodysplasia (previously myositis) ossificans progressiva

The first time a bisphosphonate was given to a human was in this disease. Despite a series of further investigations reporting positive results, it remains to be established whether this drug is really active in decreasing ectopic bone formation. Some retardation in the evolution probably occurs in many cases, but a complete standstill is rarely obtained. Lesions already formed are not influenced.

Despite this uncertainty, in view of the dismal outcome of the disease in many cases and of the lack of alternative treatment, the use of etidronate as an oral dosage of 20 mg/kg per day seems advisable. However, since this dose also inhibits mineralization of normal bone and can lead

Adverse events pp. 148–150

to rickets in children and osteomalacia in adults, and since lower doses are not effective, the drug should not be given for longer than 3 months, preferably for shorter periods of a few weeks and only when a new exacerbation occurs.

Etidronate can be tried in patients with fibrodysplasia ossificans progressiva.

Other heterotopic ossifications

Results may be somewhat more encouraging with other types of heterotopic ossification. Etidronate has been found to diminish the appearance of ossifications in patients with spinal cord injury, after cranial trauma, and after total hip replacement. In the latter, although ectopic bone formation reappears, at least partially, after discontinuation of the drug, the mobility of the hip seems nevertheless to be improved in the etidronate-treated patients. However, these results have been questioned by other authors.

Fig. 3.6-1 Effect of etidronate administered for 4 months at 20 mg daily in heterotopic ossification after placement of total hip prosthesis. (Adapted from Lowell, *et al.* (1982). In Ziegler, R. (ed.) *EHDP*, pp. 173–95. (München, Wien, Baltimore: Urban & Schwarzenberg), with copyright permission from the publisher.)

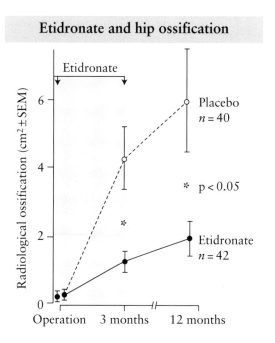

Etidronate may in some cases inhibit ectopic ossifications.

Commercially available bisphosphonates pp. 157–170

Although the efficacy of etidronate is not absolutely established, it seems nevertheless justifiable to administer it preventively in those patients who are particularly liable to develop ectopic ossifications, for example patients who require a second operation after total hip replacement because of ossifications after the first intervention. The daily oral dosage recommended by the producer is 20 mg/kg body weight, starting 1 month before the operation and given for up to 3 months after the intervention. Longer treatment should not be given, because of the possible development of osteomalacia. Etidronate is commercially available for this indication in many countries.

Etidronate appears to be useful in preventing heterotopic ossification under certain conditions. The dosage is 20 mg/kg body weight daily per os for not longer than 4 months. It is commercially available in many countries.

Conclusion

Etidronate, the only bisphosphonate investigated so far in ectopic calcification and ossification, appears to be useful for partial prevention of heterotopic ossifications in some instances. However, the effective dose is the same as that inhibiting normal mineralization, which makes the use difficult.

Recommended selected reading

Heterotopic calcification and ossification

Reviews

Thomas, B.J. (1992). Heterotopic bone formation after total hip arthroplasty. *Orthop. Clin. North Am.*, **23**, 347–58

Whyte, M.P. (1990). Extraskeletal (ectopic) calcification and ossification. In Favus, M.J. (ed.) *Primer on the Metabolic Bone Diseases and Disorders of Mineral Metabolism*, pp. 261–9. (Kelseyville, CA: American Society for Bone and Mineral Research)

Bisphosphonates, preclinical

Original articles

Fleisch, H., Russell, R.G.G., Bisaz, S., Mühlbauer, R.C. and Williams, D.A. (1970). The inhibitory effect of phosphonates on the formation of calcium phosphate crystals *in vitro* and on aortic and kidney calcification *in vivo*. *Eur. J. Clin. Invest.*, **1**, 12–18

Bisphosphonates, clinical

Reviews

Fleisch, H. (1988). Bisphosphonates: a new class of drugs in diseases of bone and calcium metabolism. In Baker, P.F. (ed.) *Handbook of Experimental Pharmacology*, vol. 83, pp. 441–66. (Berlin, Heidelberg: Springer-Verlag)

Original articles

Baumann, J.M., Bisaz, S., Fleisch, H. and Wacker, M. (1978). Biochemical and clinical effects of ethane-1-hydroxy-1,1-diphosphonate in calcium nephrolithiasis. *Clin. Sci. Mol. Med.*, **54**, 509–16

Finerman, G.A.M. and Stover, S.L. (1981). Heterotopic ossification following hip replacement or spinal cord injury. Two clinical studies with EHDP. *Metab. Bone Dis. Relat. Res.*, **4**, 337–42

Geho, W.B. and Whiteside, J.A. (1973). Experience with disodium etidronate in diseases of ectopic calcification. In Frame, B., Parfitt, A.M. and Duncan, H. (eds.) *Clinical Aspects of Metabolic Bone Disease*, pp. 506–11. (Amsterdam: Excerpta Medica)

Reiner, M., Sautter, V., Olah, A., Bossi, E., Largiadèr, U. and Fleisch, H. (1980). Diphosphonate treatment in myositis ossificans progressiva. In Caniggia, A. (ed.) *Etidronate*, pp. 237–41. (Pisa: Istituto Gentili)

Slooff, T.J.J.H., Feith, R., Bijvoet, O.L.M. and Nollen, A.J.G. (1974). The use of a disphosphonate in para-articular ossifications after total hip replacement. A clinical study. *Acta Orthop. Belg.*, **40**, 820–8

Thomas, B.J. and Amstutz, H.C. (1985). Results of the administration of diphosphonate for the prevention of heterotopic ossification after total hip arthroplasty. *J. Bone Joint Surg. (Am).*, **67**, 400–3

3.7. OTHER DISEASES

Bisphosphonates have been administered occasionally in some other diseases. Recent results indicate that pamidronate induces an improvement of bone turnover, of the radiological picture, and of pain in fibrous dysplasia of bone, a disease that presents certain histological analogies with Paget's disease, and may possibly decrease fracture incidence in osteogenesis imperfecta. Some positive results have been obtained in Sudeck's atrophy, in hereditary hyperphosphatasia, in Gaucher's disease and in diabetic Charcot neuroarthropathy. Furthermore clodronate, administered intra-articularly, has given positive results on pain and articular movement in a study in patients with osteoarthritis of the knee. The results in rheumatoid arthritis are controversial. A recent study showed a significant effect of a single infusion of pamidronate both on bone resorption and disease activity assessed by the Ritchie articular index, the number of swollen joints and also to a lesser degree, sedimentation rate and the C-reactive protein. This indication merits further investigation.

Bisphosphonates had some positive effects in fibrous dysplasia of bone, hereditary hyperphosphatasia, Gaucher's disease, diabetic Charcot neuroarthropathy, rheumatoid arthritis and, administered intra-articularly, in osteoarthritis.

Recommended selected reading

Eggelmeijer, F., Papapoulos, S.E., van Paassen, H.C., Dijkmans, B.A.C. and Breedveld, F.C. (1994). Clinical and biochemical response to single infusion of pamidronate in patients with active rheumatoid arthritis: a double blind placebo controlled study. *J. Rheumatol.*, **21**, 2016–20

Liens, D., Delmas, P.D. and Meunier, P.J. (1994). Long-term effects of intravenous pamidronate in fibrous dysplasia of bone. *Lancet*, **343**, 953–4

Samuel, R., Katz, K., Papapoulos, S.E., Yosipovitch, Z., Zaizov, R. and Liberman, U.A. (1994). Aminohydroxy propylidene bishopsphonate (APD) treatment improves the clinical skeletal manifestations of Gaucher's disease. *Pediatrics*, **94**, 385–9

Selby, P.L., Young, M.J. and Boulton, A.J.M. (1994). Bisphosphonates: a new treatment for diabetic Charcot neuroarthropathy. *Diabetic Med.*, **11**, 28–31

Singer, F., Siris, E., Shane, E., Dempster, D., Lindsay, R. and Parisien, M. (1994). Hereditary hyperphosphatasia: 20 year follow-up and response to disodium etidronate. *J. Bone Miner. Res.*, **9**, 733–8

3.8. Adverse events

3.8.1. Bisphosphonates in general

As in animals, studies in humans have revealed only a few important adverse events.

Caution must be taken with the intravenous administration of large amounts of all bisphosphonates. Rapid injection has led to renal failure, probably because of the formation of a solid phase of bisphosphonate in the blood which is then held back in the kidney. No further events of that kind have been observed since care has been taken to administer all bisphosphonates given intravenously in large amounts by slow infusion in a large volume of fluid. The exact amount of fluid necessary is not known. It is generally suggested to dilute etidronate and clodronate into at least 250 ml, 500 ml if the amount administered is large. The infusion should be slow, over at least 2 h, longer if the amount administered is high. For pamidronate 60 mg should be diluted in at least 250 ml and infused in not less than 1 h. For 90 mg the values are 500 ml and 2 h. For the more potent bisphosphonates, which are given in lower amounts, the dilution may be smaller. However, only few data exist in this respect. It has been reported that ibandronate, which is administered in a dose of only a few milligrams, can be injected in a few milliliters. For all dilutions the fluid must not contain divalent cations such as in Ringer's solution, which might form an insoluble phase with the bisphosphonate. For exact indications the package insert should be consulted.

Insoluble aggregates p. 36

When given intravenously, etidronate, clodronate and pamidronate must be diluted into 250–500 ml and infused slowly, not faster than within 2 h, longer if the amount infused is large. No data exist for the more potent compounds.

Sometimes bisphosphonates can induce a certain degree of hypocalcemia, especially when given intravenously in large amounts. This is usually without clinical effects, although occasional seizures have been described. Severe hypocalcemia has been reported in a patient who received aminoglycoside antibiotic therapy. It is possible that this was due to the incapacity of the kidneys damaged by the antibiotic to compensate for the decrease in bone resorption. Therefore, the two drugs should not be administered together.

When given orally, bisphosphonates have a tendency to produce some gastrointestinal side-effects such as nausea, dyspepsia, vomiting, gastric pain and diarrhea and sometimes even ulcerations.

> *Bisphosphonates may sometimes induce a certain degree of hypocalcemia, which is usually clinically irrelevant. An exception can be the association with aminoglycoside antibiotics with which very severe hypocalcemia can occur, so that the two drugs should not be administered together. Oral administration can be accompanied by gastrointestinal side effects.*

Kinetics
p. 58

It must be remembered that all bisphosphonates are bone seekers and therefore accumulate in the skeleton. This has the consequence that they will stay there until the bone in which they are buried is destroyed during the process of bone turnover. This can be a very long time, so that it is likely that some of the bisphosphonates may stay in the body for life. Therefore, the safety of these compounds has to be especially assured.

> *Since the bisphosphonates may stay in the body for life, their safety has to be especially assured.*

3.8.2. Individual bisphosphonates

Alendronate

Alendronate is very well tolerated up to a daily oral dose of 20 mg. At 40 mg signs of upper gastrointestinal intolerance may occur.

> *Alendronate is very well tolerated at the recommended dosage.*

Clodronate

Except for mild gastrointestinal disturbances when given orally, and one case of bronchospasm in an aspirin-sensitive patient with asthma, no proven adverse reactions have been described for clodronate. Contrary to etidronate, this compound does not inhibit mineralization of bone at the dosage used.

> *Clodronate has, except for some mild gastrointestinal disturbances when given orally, and possibly a special sensitivity in aspirin-sensitive asthma, no proven side effects.*

In the course of the clinical evaluation of this compound, some of the patients treated who had Paget's disease developed acute leukemia. This prompted the suspension of all clinical trials. Careful analysis of the data and subsequent follow-up of all the patients who had received clodronate over many years, led an *ad hoc* panel of experts to conclude that causes other than the drug, especially preselection of patients, were at least as likely or more likely than clodronate to be an explanation for the observed cases.

The suspicion that clodronate may induce leukemia has not been confirmed.

Etidronate

Etidronate has been used now in humans for more than 15 years and has proven to be very well tolerated when not administered in excessive amounts. The most common side effects of etidronate are some gastro-intestinal disturbances such as discomfort, pain and diarrhea. These occur only during oral administration and are usually of minor intensity. Most often they disappear spontaneously or can be overcome by dividing the dose.

Oral etidronate can induce gastrointestinal disturbances which are, however, mostly minor.

The major and practically only complication of treatment with etidronate is the inhibition of normal skeletal mineralization, leading to a clinical and histological picture of osteomalacia. This effect is present at daily oral doses above 800 mg and has been well documented in various conditions. The inhibition regresses after discontinuation of therapy. In Paget's disease, the picture can be that of focal osteomalacia at areas of high bone turnover and can be accompanied by the appearance of radiolucent areas. These seem to be related to bone pain. In this condition, the inhibition of mineralization has been seen at doses as low as 400 mg orally, which normally do not have this effect. The special sensitivity of patients with Paget's disease may be explained by the focal character of the disorder, leading to a high localized uptake of the drug (*see* Fig. 3.8-1).

Effect in animals pp. 52–53

Etidronate can induce focal or generalized osteomalacia when administered at high doses for periods that are too long.

Fractures have occurred in children treated for fibrodysplasia ossificans progressiva, and possibly also in adults in Paget's disease, when high doses are given over longer periods. In children, long-term treatment at an oral dose of 20 mg/kg may also induce proximal muscular weakness, leading to an abnormal gait similar to that seen in rickets.

Fibrodysplasia ossificans p. 141

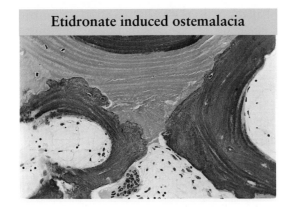

Etidronate induced ostemalacia

Fig. 3.8-1 Osteomalacia in a Pagetic patient after treatment with 20 mg/kg orally of etidronate over a long time. The dark areas are non-mineralized osteoid. (Courtesy of Dr R.K. Schenk.)

Etidronate can induce osteomalacia and rickets when given over long periods at oral doses over 10 mg/kg daily.

The effect of smaller doses in long-term therapy are more difficult to assess. A consensus exists that the intermittent treatment with 400 mg for 2 weeks every 3 months over a period of 3 years does not lead to any clinical or morphological alterations of mineralization. The situation is less clear when therapy is pursued for longer. One study showed no histological changes after 7 years, while in the large multicenter study performed in the USA, localized areas of widening of the osteoid borders suggestive of a certain degree of focal inhibition of mineralization were seen in some patients.

Inhibition of
mineralization
p. 134

The effect of very long-term treatment with 400 mg for 2 weeks every 3 months is not yet clear, but could induce some defect in mineralization.

Etidronate can cause a conspicuous rise in plasma phosphate, often to high levels, both in healthy persons and in patients. The change is associated with an increase in renal tubular reabsorption of phosphate. While it was first thought that this effect was specific for etidronate, it can also occur with tiludronate and, although very rarely, with other bisphosphonates. It is not associated with any clinical problems.

Etidronate induces an increase in plasma phosphate.

Intravenous infusions can induce a transient loss or alteration of taste with a metallic flavor which occurs, according to the package insert, in about 5% of the patients. In some individual studies the incidence was somewhat higher.

Finally, one case of bronchospasm in an aspirin-sensitive patient has been described.

Pamidronate

The intravenous administration of pamidronate induces on the average in about 10% of the patients, but in some trials more often, a transient pyrexia of usually 1–2 °C, sometimes more. Occasionally it is accompanied by pain in the bones. It is maximal within 24–48 h and disappears within approximately 3 days, even when treatment is continued. The effect is dose-dependent and is usually only observed once, even if treatment is discontinued and restarted later. The pyrexia is accompanied by a decrease in peripheral lymphocytes, an increase in serum C-reactive protein and a decrease in serum zinc. The mechanism of these changes, which resemble an acute-phase response, is still not completely understood, but seems to involve the stimulation of macrophages to release IL-6, which increases in plasma. This event occurs also with some other aminobisphosphonates, but not with etidronate and clodronate. Up to now no negative consequences of these episodes have been described, and these appear to bear no clinical relevance, except for the slight discomfort in the first days of treatment.

> ***Pamidronate, like some other aminobisphosphonates, induces transient pyrexia in the course of an acute-phase-like reaction.***

Pamidronate administered intravenously can induce occasional local thrombophlebitis at the infusion site. Otherwise it is well tolerated when given through this route. Recently it has, however, been reported that in patients with Paget's disease who received pamidronate intravenously at doses equal to or higher than 30 mg a week for 6 continuous weeks, four out of ten have displayed a defect in mineralization in both Pagetic and normal bone. Furthermore, patients who had received 45 mg intravenously every 3 months for 1 year displayed osteoid borders larger than normal. These changes disappeared after cessation of treatment. In another study, a child with fibrous dysplasia, who was given 60 mg daily intravenously of pamidronate for 3 days in a continuous infusion every 6 months over 18 months, developed a radiological picture of defective mineralization of the epiphyseal plate, but without other clinical consequences.

> *Pamidronate administered at intravenous doses equal to or higher than 180 mg/year can induce a transient inhibition of mineralization.*

When given orally at doses of 300 mg or more daily, pamidronate can induce gastrointestinal disturbances with nausea, vomiting, pain and diarrhea. Some cases of erosive esophagitis have also been reported. At 300 mg the effect seems to depend upon the study. The occurrence of these effects, which are not limited to pamidronate only but occur also to some extent with other aminobisphosphonates, varies greatly from study to study. They were reported mostly but not only in patients with tumor bone disease who may be more sensitive than other patients and who are often given higher doses. The heterogeneity of the response also suggests that the formulation may be crucial, since this has varied a great deal between the studies. The timing of the dose is relevant, and it is important to avoid administration before sleeping, especially in bedridden patients. Finally, the amount of fluid given with the drug is of importance, and it is advised to take it with sufficient liquid, about 150 ml. With these various points taken into account and with the use of enterocoated micropellet capsules, these gastrointestinal side effects may be diminished in the future. However, in the current trials, the dose of 300 mg is not exceeded.

> *Oral pamidronate as well as other aminobisphosphonates can give rise to dose-related gastrointestinal disturbances that may be severe.*

Recently the producer reported that on rare occasions, ocular adverse reactions occurred, which recurred under rechallenging, in patients receiving intravenous pamidronate. These reactions included anterior uveitis, episcleritis or scleritis, and conjunctivitis.

> *Pamidronate can in rare cases induce ocular adverse reactions.*

Tiludronate

Tiludronate appears to be well tolerated. One patient with a personal and family history of allergies was reported to have developed a widespread erythematous skin condition with vesicular and vesiculobullous periphery and a histological picture of epidermal necrosis. The mucous membranes remained unaffected. The condition was diagnosed at first as toxicoderma, later possibly as pemphigus, and required systemic corticosteroid therapy.

Diminution of renal function has been described in tumor-induced hypercalcemia with a high dose of an intravenous formulation, but the interpretation of these data is difficult, in view of the severe condition of the patients treated.

Other bisphosphonates

No data are yet available.

Recommended selected reading

Original articles

Etidronate

Bounameaux, H.M., Schifferli, J., Montani, J.P., Jung, A. and Chatelanat, F. (1983). Renal failure associated with intravenous diphosphonate (letter). *Lancet*, **1**, 471

Boyce, B.F., Smith, L., Fogelman, I., Johnston, E., Ralston, S. and Boyle, I.T. (1984). Focal osteomalacia due to low-dose diphosphonate therapy in Paget's disease. *Lancet*, **1**, 821–4

de Vries, H.R. and Bijvoet, O.L.M. (1974). Results of prolonged treatment of Paget's disease of bone with disodium ethane-1-hydroxy-1,1-diphosphonate (EHDP). *Neth. J. Med.*, **17**, 281–98

Jowsey, J., Riggs, B.L., Kelly, P.J., Hoffman, D.L. and Bordier, P. (1971). The treatment of osteoporosis with disodium ethane-1-hydroxy-1,1-diphosphonate. *J. Lab. Clin. Med.*, **78**, 574–84

Khairi, M.R.A., Altman, R.D., DeRosa, G.P., Zimmermann, J., Schenk, R.K. and Johnston, C.C. (1977). Sodium etidronate in the treatment of Paget's disease of bone. A study of long-term results. *Ann. Intern. Med.*, **87**, 656–63

Nagant de Deuxchaisnes, C., Rombouts-Lindemans, C., Huaux, J.P., Devogelaer, J.P., Malghem, J., Maldague, B., Withofs, H. and Meersseman, F. (1981). Paget's disease of bone. *Br. Med. J.*, **283**, 1054–5

Recker, R.R., Hassing, G.S., Lau, J.R. and Saville, P.D. (1973). The hyperphosphatemic effect of disodium ethane-1-hydroxy-1,1-diphosphonate (EHDP^{TM}): renal handling of phosphorus and the renal response to parathyroid hormone. *J. Lab. Clin. Med.*, **81**, 258–66

Reiner, M., Sautter, V., Olah, A., Bossi, E., Largiadèr, U. and Fleisch, H. (1980). Diphosphonate treatment in myositis ossificans progressiva. In Caniggia, A. (ed.) *Etidronate*, pp. 237–41. (Pisa: Istituto Gentili)

Rolla, G., Bucca, C. and Brussino, L. (1994). Bisphosphonate-induced bronchoconstriction in aspirin-sensitive asthma. *Lancet*, **343**, 426–7

Clodronate

Pedersen-Bjergaard, U. and Myhre, J. (1991). Severe hypoglycaemia after treatment with diphosphonate and aminoglycoside. *Br. Med. J.*, **302**, 295

Adverse events

Rolla, G., Bucca, C. and Brussino, L. (1994). Bisphosphonate-induced broncoconstriction in aspirin-sensitive asthma. *Lancet*, **343**, 426–7

Pamidronate

Adami, S., Bhalla, A.K., Dorizzi, R., Montesanti, F., Rosini, S., Salvagno, G. and Lo Cascio, V. (1987). The acute-phase response after bisphosphonate administration. *Calcif. Tissue Int.*, **41**, 326–31

Adamson, B.B., Gallacher, S.J., Byars, J., Ralston, S.H., Boyle, J.T. and Boyce, B.F. (1993). Mineralisation defects with pamidronate therapy for Paget's disease. *Lancet*, **342**, 1459–60

Dodwell, D.J., Howell, A. and Ford, J. (1990). Reduction in calcium excretion in women with breast cancer and bone metastases using the oral bisphosphonate pamidronate. *Br. J. Cancer*, **61**, 123–5

Harinck, H.I.J., Papapoulos, S.E., Blanksma, H.J., Moolenaar, A.J., Vermeij, P. and Bijvoet, O.L.M. (1987). Paget's disease of bone: early and late responses to three different modes of treatment with aminohydroxypropylidene bisphosphonate (APD). *Br. Med. J.*, **295**, 1301–5

Liens, D., Delmas, P.D. and Meunier, P.J. (1994). Long-term effects of intravenous pamidronate in fibrous dysplasia of bone. *Lancet*, **343**, 953–4

Lufkin, E.G., Argueta, R., Whitaker, M.D., Cameron, A.L., Wong, V.H., Egan, K.S., O'Fallon, W.M. and Riggs, B.L. (1994). Pamidronate: an unrecognized problem in gastrointestinal tolerability. *Osteoporosis Int.*, **4**, 320–2

Marcarol, V. and Fraunfelder, F.T. (1994). Pamidronate disodium and possible ocular adverse drug reactions. *Am. J. Opthalmol.*, **118**, 220–4

Schweitzer, D.H. and Oostendorp-van de Ruit, M., van der Pluijm, G., Löwik, C.W.G.M. and Papapoulos, S.E. (1995). Interleukin-6 and the acute phase response during treatment of patients with Paget's disease with the nitrogen-containing bisphosphonate dimethylaminohydroxypropylidene bisphosphonate. *J. Bone Miner. Res.*, **10**, 956–62

van Breukelen, F.J.M., Bijvoet, O.L.M., Frijlink, W.B., Sleeboom, H.P., Mulder, H. and van Oosterom, A.T. (1982). Efficacy of amino-hydroxypropylidene bisphosphonate in hypercalcemia: observations on regulation of serum calcium. *Calcif. Tissue Int.*, **34**, 321–7

van Holten-Verzantvoort, A.T., Bijvoet, O.L.M., Cleton, F.J., Hermans, J., Kroon, H.M., Harinck, H.I.J., Vermey, P., Elte, J.W.F., Neijt, J.P., Beex, L.V.A.M. and Blijham, G. (1987). Reduced morbidity from skeletal metastases in breast cancer patients during long-term bisphosphonate (APD) treatment. *Lancet*, **2**, 983–5

Tiludronate

Dumon, J.C., Magritte, A. and Body, J.J. (1991). Efficacy and safety of the bisphosphonate tiludronate for the treatment of tumor-associated hypercalcemia. *Bone Miner.*, **15**, 257–66

Roux, C., Listrat, V., Villette, B., Lessana-Leibowitch, M., Ethgen, D., Pelissier, C., Dougados, M. and Amor, B. (1992). Long-lasting dermatological lesions after tiludronate therapy. *Calcif. Tissue Int.*, **50**, 378–80

3.9. CONTRAINDICATIONS

Up to now no contraindications have been described for the bisphosphonates. The question is often raised whether these compounds can be administered in renal failure. Since they are cleared from blood to a large extent by the skeleton, there is no theoretical reason to renounce bisphosphonates in patients with moderate renal failure. Pamidronate has in fact been administered successfully to treat hypercalcemia in patients with renal failure. However, plasma levels are likely to be higher, so that the dose should be reduced. The exact amount of this reduction will only be known when plasma data are available. In the meantime it is suggested to decrease the dosage up to a quarter of the amount recommended, according to the degree of renal failure. In addition, a certain caution may be indicated with etidronate, because of its propensity to increase phosphatemia, which is already high in renal failure.

Kinetics p. 58

There is no absolute contraindication to the use of bisphosphonates in renal failure.

Another open question is whether bisphosphonates can be given during fracture healing or during stabilization of orthopedic implants such as hip prostheses. Recent data indicate that at least clodronate and pamidronate do not significantly hamper fracture healing in the rat. On the contrary the callus can be thicker, contain more calcium and have greater mechanical strength but is remodeled at a later stage to normal bone size. Furthermore this bisphosphonate can prevent bone loss under the plate. It would appear, therefore, that there is no contraindication with the low doses such as those used in osteoporosis and which do not inhibit mineralization. In contrast, large doses of etidronate, which are likely to inhibit mineralization, should be avoided.

Inhibition of mineralization pp. 148–149

Fracture healing or fresh orthopedic implants are no contraindication to the use of bisphosphonates, provided they are not given in doses that inhibit mineralization.

In view of the gastrointestinal effects of bisphosphonates during oral administration, caution should be used when giving these compounds, especially pamidronate, orally to patients with gastrointestinal disorders such as ulcers.

Gastrointestinal effects p. 151

Oral administration should be used with caution in patients with inflammatory gastrointestinal conditions.

Effect on fetus
p. 65

Since bisphosphonates can cross the placenta and can have deleterious effects on the fetus when given in high doses, they should not be used in pregnant women. Furthermore, since it is not known whether they are excreted in milk, it is also not advisable to give them to lactating women.

> ***Bisphosphonates should not be given during pregnancy and lactation.***

Adverse
events
p. 146

Few data are available on inter-relations with other drugs. Bisphosphonates should not be administered with aminoglycoside antibiotics, because of the appearance of hypocalcemia. No data are available on the effect of the simultaneous administration of different bisphosphonates. Therefore, only one bisphosphonate should be administered at a time.

> ***A bisphosphonate should not be given together with another compound of the same class and with aminoglycosides.***

Recommended selected reading

Goodship, A.E., Walker, P.C., McNally, D., Chambers, T. and Green, J.R. (1994). Use of a bisphosphonate (pamidronate) to modulate fracture repair in ovine bone. *Ann. Oncol.*, **5**, (Suppl. 7), S53–S55

Nyman, M.T., Paavolainen, P. and Lindholm, T.S. (1993). Clodronate increases the calcium content in fracture callus. An experimental study in rats. *Arch. Orthop. Trauma Surg.*, **112**, 228–31

Tarvainen, R., Olkkonen, H., Nevalainen, T., Hyvönen, P., Arnala, I. and Alhava, E. (1994). Effect of clodronate on fracture healing in denervated rats. *Bone*, **6**, 701–5

3.10. FUTURE PROSPECTS

The bisphosphonates present a most interesting development in the field of treatment of bone diseases, and it is probable that we are only at the beginning of a new area of therapy.

Many issues are still unresolved. For example, we do not yet know whether we have found the optimal regimen for the compounds available. This is especially the case in treatment of osteoporosis. Is there an advantage to the use of an intermittent therapy, as is proposed for etidronate? If so, which would be the optimal regimen? Could one think of a longer, possibly even yearly treatment interval?

Although the differences between the various bisphosphonates appear to be more quantitative than qualitative, it might nevertheless be possible in the future to synthesize compounds that have certain specific effects. For example, a compound acting only on ectopic calcification would be most useful.

Since the long persistence of bisphosphonates in the body is a concern for some, it may be possible in the future to devise drugs that are similar to the bisphosphonates, have similar effects, but are metabolically broken down.

The possible use of bisphosphonates in diseases other than those of bone has not yet been practically investigated. The results on experimental arthritis are most encouraging in this respect. Another interesting application may be in the dental field.

In addition, the use of bisphosphonates or bisphosphonate analogs as carriers for drugs to be brought to the bone or to other calcified tissues is another line of investigation.

Lastly, it could be that with a better knowledge of the mode of action of these compounds at the cellular level, new insight will be gained into the physiological and pathophysiological function of bone, opening up new approaches to therapy.

4. Commercially available bisphosphonates

Country				
Bisphosphonate	Trade name	Company	Indications	Form
Argentina				
Alendronate	Fosamax	Merck Sharp & Dohme	Postmenopausal osteoporosis	po
Clodronate	Ostac	Boehringer Mannheim	Tumoral osteolysis Hypercalcemia of malignancy	po & iv
Pamidronate	Aminomux	Gador	Paget's disease Osteoporosis	po
			Tumoral osteolysis Hypercalcemia of malignancy	iv
Australia				
Etidronate	Didronel	Procter & Gamble	Paget's disease Heterotopic ossification	po
	Didrocal		Osteoporosis	
Pamidronate	Aredia	Ciba-Geigy	Hypercalcemia of malignancy	iv
Austria				
Clodronate	Bonefos	Laevosan	Hypercalcemia of malignancy Tumoral osteolysis	po & iv
	Lodronat	Boehringer Mannheim	Hypercalcemia of malignancy Tumoral osteolysis	po & iv

continued

| Country | | | | |
Bisphosphonate	Trade name	Company	Indications	Form
Etidronate	Didronel	Procter & Gamble	Paget's disease Heterotopic 71ossification	po
		Rhoem Pharma	Osteoporosis	
Pamidronate	Aredia	Ciba-Geigy	Hypercalcemia of malignancy Tumoral osteolysis	iv
Bahrein				
Clodronate	Bonefos	Maskati Pharmacy	Hypercalcemia of malignancy	po & iv
	Ostac	Boehringer Mannheim/ Forooghi Pharmacy	Hypercalcemia of malignancy Tumoral osteolysis	po & iv
Belgium				
Clodronate	Bonefos	UCB	Hypercalcemia of malignancy Tumoral osteolysis Osteolytic bone metastases	po & iv
Etidronate	Didronel	Procter & Gamble	Hypercalcemia of malignancy	iv
			Paget's disease Periarticular ossification	po
	Osteodidronel		Osteoporosis	
Pamidronate	Aredia	Ciba-Geigy	Hypercalcemia of malignancy	iv
Brazil				
Clodronate	Ostac	Asta Medica	Hypercalcemia of malignancy Bone metastases	po & iv
Pamidronate	Aredia	Ciba-Geigy	Hypercalcemia of malignancy Bone metastases	iv
Canada				
Clodronate	Bonefos	Rhône-Poulenc Rorer	Hypercalcemia of malignancy	po & iv
	Ostac	Boehringer Mannheim	Hypercalcemia of malignancy	po & iv
Etidronate	Didronel	Procter & Gamble	Paget's disease	po

continued

Country				
Bisphosphonate	Trade name	Company	Indications	Form
		Knoll	Hypercalcemia of malignancy	iv
Pamidronate	Aredia	Ciba-Geigy	Hypercalcemia of malignancy Paget's disease	iv
Chile				
Clodronate	Bonefos	Leiras	Hypercalcemia of malignancy Paget's disease	po & iv
	Ostac	Boehringer Mannheim	Hypercalcemia of malignancy Paget's disease	po & iv
P.R. China				
Clodronate	Bonefos	MRL Corp. Ltd.	Tumoral osteolysis	po & iv
Columbia				
Clodronate	Ostac	Boehringer Mannheim	Hypercalcemia of malignancy	iv
		Grünenthal	Paget's disease	iv
Costa Rica				
Alendronate	Fosamax	Merck Sharp & Dohme	Postmenopausal osteoporosis	po
Cyprus				
Clodronate	Ostac	Papaellina	Hypercalcemia of malignancy Tumoral osteolysis	po & iv
Czech Republic				
Clodronate	Bonefos	Leiras	Tumoral osteolysis	po & iv
	Lodronat	Boehringer Mannheim	Tumoral osteolysis	po & iv
Pamidronate	Aredia	Ciba-Geigy	Hypercalcemia of malignancy Tumoral osteolysis Bone metastases	iv
Denmark				
Alendronate	Fosamax	Merck Sharp & Dohme	Postmenopausal osteoporosis	po

continued

Country				
Bisphosphonate	Trade name	Company	Indications	Form
Clodronate	Bonefos	Astra	Hypercalcemia of malignancy Tumoral osteolysis	po & iv
	Ostac	Ercopharm	Hypercalcemia of malignancy Tumoral osteolysis	po & iv
Etidronate	Didronate	Roche	Paget's disease Heterotopic ossification Osteoporosis	po
Pamidronate	Aredia	Ciba-Geigy	Hypercalcemia of malignancy	iv
Dominican Republic				
Clodronate	Ostac	Boehringer Mannheim	Hypercalcemia of malignancy Tumoral osteolysis	po & iv
Ecuador				
Clodronate	Ostac	Grünenthal	Hypercalcemia of malignancy Tumoral osteolysis	po & iv
El Salvador				
Alendronate	Fosamax	Merck Sharp & Dohme	Postmenopausal osteoporosis	po
Clodronate	Ostac	Boehringer Mannheim	Hypercalcemia of malignancy Tumoral osteolysis	po & iv
Pamidronate	Aminomux	Marco-Med	Paget's disease Osteoporosis	po
Estonia				
Clodronate	Bonefos	Leiras	Tumoral osteolysis	po & iv
Finland				
Clodronate	Bonefos	Leiras	Hypercalcemia of malignancy Tumoral osteolysis Osteolytic bone metastases	po & iv
Etidronate	Didronel	Procter & Gamble	Special license	po & iv
Pamidronate	Aredia	Ciba-Geigy	Hypercalcemia of malignancy	iv

continued

Commercial index

Country Bisphosphonate	Trade name	Company	Indications	Form
France				
Clodronate	Clastoban	Roger Bellon	Hypercalcemia of malignancy Tumoral osteolysis	po & iv
	Lytos	Boehringer Mannheim	Hypercalcemia of malignancy Tumoral osteolysis	po & iv
Etidronate	Didronel	Procter & Gamble	Paget's disease Osteoporosis Hypercalcemia of malignancy	po iv
Pamidronate	Aredia	Ciba-Geigy	Hypercalcemia of malignancy	iv
Tiludronate	Skelid	Sanofi Winthrop	Paget's disease	po
Germany				
Clodronate	Bonefos	Astra	Hypercalcemia of malignancy Tumoral osteolysis	po & iv
	Ostac	Boehringer Mannheim	Hypercalcemia of malignancy Tumoral osteolysis	po & iv
Etidronate	Diphos Etidronate iv	Roehm Pharma	Paget's disease Heterotopic ossification Hypercalcemia of malignancy	po iv
Pamidronate	Aredia	Ciba-Geigy	Hypercalcemia of malignancy	iv
Greece				
Clodronate	Bonefos	Leiras	Tumoral osteolysis	po & iv
	Ostac	Farmalex	Hypercalcemia of malignancy Tumoral osteolysis Paget's disease	po & iv
Etidronate	Ostopor	Unipharm	Osteoporosis	po
Pamidronate	Aredia	Ciba-Geigy	Hypercalcemia of malignancy	iv
Guatemala				
Alendronate	Fosamax	Merck Sharp & Dohme	Postmenopausal osteoporosis	po

continued

Country				
Bisphosphonate	Trade name	Company	Indications	Form
Clodronate	Ostac	Boehringer Mannheim	Hypercalcemia of malignancy Tumoral osteolysis	po & iv
Honduras				
Alendronate	Fosamax	Merck Sharp & Dohme	Postmenopausal osteoporosis	po
Clodronate	Ostac	Boehringer Mannheim	Hypercalcemia of malignancy Tumoral osteolysis	po & iv
Hong Kong				
Clodronate	Bonefos	MRL Corp. Ltd.	Hypercalcemia of malignancy Tumoral osteolysis	po & iv
	Ostac	Boehringer Mannheim	Hypercalcemia of malignancy Tumoral osteolysis	po & iv
Pamidronate	Aredia	Ciba-Geigy	Hypercalcemia of malignancy	iv
Hungary				
Clodronate	Bonefos	Leiras	Hypercalcemia of malignancy Tumoral osteolysis	po & iv
	Lodronat	Boehringer Mannheim	Hypercalcemia of malignancy Tumoral osteolysis	po & iv
Iceland				
Clodronate	Bonefos	Asgeir Sigurdsson	Hypercalcemia of malignancy Tumoral osteolysis	po & iv
	Loron	Ercopharm	Hypercalcemia of malignancy Tumoral osteolysis	po & iv
Pamidronate	Aredia	Ciba-Geigy	Hypercalcemia of malignancy	iv
India				
Pamidronate	Aminomux	Mac Laboratories	Hypercalcemia of malignancy	iv
Indonesia				
Clodronate	Bonefos	Pt Djaja Bimaagung	Hypercalcemia of malignancy Tumoral osteolysis	po & iv

continued

Country				
Bisphosphonate	**Trade name**	**Company**	**Indications**	**Form**
	Ostac	Boehringer Mannheim	Hypercalcemia of malignancy Tumoral osteolysis	po & iv
Ireland				
Etidronate	Didronel	Procter & Gamble	Paget's disease Heterotopic ossification Hypercalcemia of malignancy	po iv
Clodronate	Bonefos	Boehringer Ingelheim	Hypercalcemia of malignancy Tumoral osteolysis	po & iv
Pamidronate	Aredia	Ciba-Geigy	Hypercalcemia of malignancy Tumoral osteolysis	iv
Israel				
Clodronate	Bonefos	Chiminter	Hypercalcemia of malignancy Tumoral osteolysis	po & iv
	Ostac	Abic	Hypercalcemia of malignancy Tumoral osteolysis	po & iv
Pamidronate	Aredia	Ciba-Geigy	Hypercalcemia of malignancy	iv
Italy				
Alendronate	Adronat	Neopharmed	Osteoporosis	po
	Alendros	Gentili	Osteoporosis	po
	Dronal	Sigma-Tau	Osteoporosis	po
	Fosamax	MSD	Osteoporosis	po
Clodronate	Clasteon	Gentili	Tumoral osteolysis Myeloma Primary hyperparathyroidism Osteoporosis	po, iv & im po
	Difosfonal	SPA	Tumoral osteolysis Myeloma Primary hyperparathyroidism Osteoporosis	po, iv & im po
	Ossiten	Boehringer Mannheim	Hypercalcemia of malignancy Tumoral osteolysis Osteoporosis	po & iv po
Etidronate	Etidron	Gentili	Paget's disease	po

continued

Country Bisphosphonate	Trade name	Company	Indications	Form
	Didrokit	Procter & Gamble	Osteoporosis	po
Pamidronate	Aredia	Ciba-Geigy	Hypercalcemia of malignancy	iv
Japan				
Etidronate	Didronel	Sumitomo	Paget's disease Heterotopic ossification	po
Pamidronate	Aredia	Ciba-Geigy	Hypercalcemia of malignancy	iv
Jordan				
Clodronate	Bonefos	The Arab Drug Store	Tumoral osteolysis Hypercalcemia of malignancy	po & iv
Khasakstan				
Alendronate	Fosamax	Merck Sharp & Dohme	Postmenopausal osteoporosis	po
Korea				
Clodronate	Ostac	CKD	Hypercalcemia of malignancy Tumoral osteolysis	po & iv
Kuwait				
Clodronate	Bonefos	Warba Medical Supplies	Paget's disease Hypercalcemia of malignancy Tumoral osteolysis	po & iv
	Ostac	Boehringer Mannheim/ Al-Ghanim	Hypercalcemia of malignancy Tumoral osteolysis	po & iv
Luxemburg				
Clodronate	Ostac	Boehringer Mannheim	Hypercalcemia of malignancy Tumoral osteolysis	po & iv
Etidronate	Didronel	Procter & Gamble	Paget's disease Hypercalcemia of malignancy	po iv
Pamidronate	Aredia	Ciba-Geigy	Hypercalcemia of malignancy	iv

continued

Commercial index

Country				
Bisphosphonate	Trade name	Company	Indications	Form
Malaysia				
Clodronate	Bonefos	Waleta Malaysia Son BHD	Tumoral osteolysis	po & iv
	Ostac	Boehringer Mannheim	Tumoral bone disease	po & iv
Malta				
Clodronate	Ostac	Vivian	Hypercalcemia of malignancy Tumoral osteolysis	po & iv
Mexico				
Alendronate	Fosamax	Merck	Osteoporosis	po
Pamidronate	Aredia	Ciba-Geigy	Bone metastases	iv
Morocco				
Etidronate	Didronel	Société Marocaine des Produits Bottu	Osteoporosis	po
The Netherlands				
Clodronate	Bonefos	Taicoms Trading Co.	Hypercalcemia of malignancy	po & iv
	Ostac	Boehringer Mannheim	Hypercalcemia of malignancy	po & iv
Etidronate	Didrokit Didronel	Procter & Gamble	Osteoporosis Paget's disease Heterotopic ossification Hypercalcemia of malignancy	po iv
Pamidronate	Aredia	Ciba-Geigy	Hypercalcemia of malignancy	iv
New Zealand				
Etidronate	Didronel	Pharmaco (NZ)	Paget's disease Heterotopic ossification Osteoporosis Hypercalcemia of malignancy	po iv
Clodronate	Ostac	Boehringer Mannheim	Tumoral osteolysis	po
Pamidronate	Aredia	Ciba-Geigy	Hypercalcemia of malignancy Tumoral osteolysis Bone metastases Paget's disease	iv

continued

Country				
Bisphosphonate	Trade name	Company	Indications	Form
Norway				
Clodronate	Bonefos	Leiras	Hypercalcemia of malignancy	po & iv
	Ostac	Organon	Hypercalcemia of malignancy	po & iv
Etidronate	Didronel	Procter & Gamble	Special license	po & iv
Pamidronate	Aredia	Ciba-Geigy	Hypercalcemia of malignancy	iv
Oman				
Clodronate	Bonefos	Oriental Pharmacy	Tumoral osteolysis	po & iv
Pakistan				
Clodronate	Bonefos	Leiras	Tumoral osteolysis	po & iv
Panama				
Alendronate	Fosamax	Merck Sharp & Dohme	Postmenopausal osteoporosis	po
Clodronate	Ostac	Quimifar	Hypercalcemia of malignancy Tumoral osteolysis	po & iv
Peru				
Alendronate	Fosamax	Merck	Osteoporosis	po
Philippines				
Clodronate	Bonefos	Rhône-Poulenc Rorer	Paget's disease Hypercalcemia of malignancy Tumoral osteolysis	po & iv
Poland				
Clodronate	Bonefos	Leiras	Tumoral osteolysis	po & iv
	Lodronat	Boehringer Mannheim	Tumoral osteolysis	po & iv
Pamidronate	Aredia	Ciba-Geigy	Hypercalcemia of malignancy Bone metastases Paget's disease	iv

continued

Country				
Bisphosphonate	Trade name	Company	Indications	Form
Portugal				
Clodronate	Ostac	Boehringer Mannheim	Hypercalcemia of malignancy Tumoral osteolysis	po & iv
Etidronate	Didronel	Lab Normal	Paget's disease Heterotopic ossification Osteoporosis	po
Pamidronate	Aredia	Ciba-Geigy	Hypercalcemia of malignancy Tumoral osteolysis	iv
Quatar				
Clodronate	Ostac	Boehringer Mannheim Opsis Pharmacy	Hypercalcemia of malignancy Tumoral osteolysis	po & iv
Russia				
Clodronate	Bonefos	Leiras	Hypercalcemia of malignancy Tumoral osteolysis	po & iv
Saudi-Arabia				
Clodronate	Bonefos	Leiras	Hypercalcemia of malignancy Tumoral osteolysis	po & iv
Singapore				
Clodronate	Bonefos	Inchcape Healthcare Pharmaceutical Division	Hypercalcemia of malignancy Tumoral osteolysis	po & iv
	Ostac	Boehringer Mannheim	Hypercalcemia of malignancy Tumoral osteolysis	po & iv
Pamidronate	Aredia	Ciba-Geigy	Hypercalcemia of malignancy	iv
Slovakia				
Clodronate	Bonefos	Leiras	Hypercalcemia of malignancy Tumoral osteolysis Osteolytic metastases	po & iv
	Lodronat	Boehringer Mannheim	Hypercalcemia of malignancy Tumoral osteolysis	po & iv

continued

Country *Bisphosphonate*	Trade name	Company	Indications	Form
Pamidronate	Aredia	Ciba-Geigy	Hypercalcemia of malignancy Tumoral osteolysis	iv
Slovenia				
Clodronate	Lodronat	Boehringer Mannheim	Hypercalcemia of malignancy Tumoral osteolysis	po & iv
South Africa				
Clodronate	Ostac	Boehringer Mannheim	Hypercalcemia of malignancy	po & iv
Pamidronate	Aredia	Ciba-Geigy	Hypercalcemia of malignancy	iv
Spain				
Clodronate	Bonefos	Boehringer Ingelheim	Hypercalcemia of malignancy Tumoral osteolysis	po & iv
	Mebonat	Boehringer Mannheim	Hypercalcemia of malignancy Tumoral osteolysis	po & iv
Etidronate	Difosphen/Osteum	Rubio/Vinas	Osteoporosis	po
Sri Lanka				
Clodronate	Ostac	J. L. Morison	Hypercalcemia of malignancy Tumoral osteolysis	po & iv
Sweden				
Alendronate	Fosamax	Merck Sharp & Dohme	Postmenopausal osteoporosis	po
Clodronate	Bonefos	Astra	Hypercalcemia of malignancy Tumoral osteolysis	po & iv
	Ostac	Boehringer Mannheim	Hypercalcemia of malignancy Tumoral osteolysis	po & iv
Etidronate	Didronate	Roche	Paget's disease Heterotopic ossification Osteoporosis	po
Pamidronate	Aredia	Ciba-Geigy	Hypercalcemia of malignancy	iv

continued

Country Bisphosphonate	Trade name	Company	Indications	Form
Switzerland				
Clodronate	Bonefos	Astra	Hypercalcemia of malignancy Tumoral osteolysis	po & iv
	Ostac	Boehringer Mannheim	Hypercalcemia of malignancy Tumoral osteolysis	po & iv
Etidronate	Didronel	Procter & Gamble	Paget's disease Heterotopic ossification	po
Pamidronate	Aredia	Ciba-Geigy	Hypercalcemia of malignancy	iv
Tiludronate	Skelid	Sanofi Winthrop	Paget's disease	po
Taiwan				
Clodronate	Bonefos	Leiras	Hypercalcemia of malignancy Tumoral osteolysis	po & iv
Thailand				
Clodronate	Bonefos	Berli Jucker Co. Ltd.	Hypercalcemia of malignancy Tumoral osteolysis	po & iv
Ukraine				
Alendronate	Fosamax	Merck Sharp & Dohme	Postmenopausal osteoporosis	po
United Arab Emirates				
Clodronate	Bonefos	Leiras	Hypercalcemia of malignancy Tumoral osteolysis	po & iv
	Ostac	Boehringer Mannheim Pharmatrade	Hypercalcemia of malignancy Tumoral osteolysis	po & iv
United Kingdom				
Clodronate	Bonefos	Boehringer Ingelheim	Hypercalcemia of malignancy Tumoral osteolysis	po & iv
	Loron	Boehringer Mannheim	Hypercalcemia of malignancy Tumoral osteolysis	po & iv
Etidronate	Didronel PMO	Procter & Gamble	Paget's disease Heterotopic ossification Osteoporosis	po

continued

Country				
Bisphosphonate	Trade name	Company	Indications	Form
			Hypercalcemia of malignancy	iv
Pamidronate	Aredia	Ciba-Geigy	Hypercalcemia of malignancy	iv
United States				
Etidronate	Didronel	Procter & Gamble	Paget's disease Heterotopic ossification	po
		MGI Pharma	Hypercalcemia of malignancy	iv
Pamidronate	Aredia	Ciba-Geigy	Hypercalcemia of malignancy Paget's disease	iv
Uruguay				
Pamidronate	Aminomux	Gador	Paget's disease Osteoporosis	po
			Tumoral osteolysis Hypercalcemia of malignancy	iv
Venezuela				
Clodronate	Ostac	Laboratorios Vargas	Hypercalcemia of malignancy Tumoral osteolysis	po & iv

This list is based upon information received from the companies mentioned in it. It is possible that we missed some firms selling bisphosphonates and of which we were not aware. If this was the case, we are sorry for the unintentional omission.

October 1995

Index

172